ALTERNATIVE THERAPIES

Alternative Therapies

Earle Weisenburger
& Irvin Boichuk

oolichan books
LANTZVILLE / BRITISH COLUMBIA / CANADA
1996

Canadian Cataloguing in Publication Data

Weisenburger, Earle, 1943-
    Alternative therapies for cancer & arthritis

    Includes bibliographical references and index.
    ISBN O-88982-154-2

    1. Cancer—Alternative treatment. 2. Arthritis—Alternative
treatment. I. Boichuk, Irv, 1948- II. Title.
    RC271.A62W44 1995   616.99'406   C95-911012-7

The cover illustration represents the inner sanctuary where one
can find peace and healing. The sanctuary shines both within
and without. The bird's wings are lifted in flight, yet the head
is curved in a position of rest. This is a reproduction of an original work of art by Signy Cohen, Box 441, Tofino, B.C. Signy
owns her own art gallery in Tofino. Her work is drawn on hand-
engraved paper using coloured pencils, providing a unique tex-
ture and depth. The publisher and authors wish to thank Signy
Cohen for permission to reproduce her work.

The publisher gratefully acknowledges the assistance of the
Canada Council.

Published by
Oolichan Books, Box 10, Lantzville, British Columbia
Canada V0R 2H0

Printed in Canada by Hignell Printing Limited
Winnipeg, Manitoba

CONTENTS

Preface   vii

About the Authors   viii

Introduction   ix

Chapter 1 / Alternatives   13

Chapter 2 / Clinic Therapies   25

Chapter 3 / Chemical Therapies   51

Chapter 4 / Dietary Therapies   69

Chapter 5 / Herbal Therapies   87

Chapter 6 / Miscellaneous Therapies   115

Notes   131

Index   139

Disclaimer

This publication has been developed both for the general public and to assist physicians in providing information to patients. The views and ideas presented in this book should not be interpreted as being the official policy of the publisher nor of the authors. The data within is presented as being the most accurate and informative available. Neither the author nor the publisher assumes responsibility for or endorses the views of source information.

Preface

We researched and developed this book as a guide to alternative therapies for cancer and arthritis. When other applications for the therapies showed up in the research, we included them as well. For additional reading, the sources of information may be located in the references at the end of this book.

Dr. Earle Weisenburger provided definitions and explanations to assist those not familiar with medical and scientific terminology. This information is found enclosed in brackets throughout the text.

We also researched much additional information, such as regulations, descriptions of plants, and compositions of chemical and herbal therapies.

This book provides neither approval nor disapproval of any type of therapy. The intent is to provide an understanding of those therapies that are currently available. We hope to present sufficient information to let the reader make an informed choice.

We strongly recommend that you consult with your physician before attempting any unconventional therapy. As you read this book you will note that many of the alternative therapies described are not without serious, even fatal side effects. You should not expect to find that the promotional material and labels provide appropriate warnings.

Neither the publisher nor the author accepts responsibility for claims for or against any treatment or therapy contained in this book, nor for any statements by quoted authors.

About the Authors

Dr. Earle Weisenburger graduated in medicine from the University of Alberta, Edmonton, Canada. He has been in general practice in Nanaimo, British Columbia for the past twenty years. He became interested in alternative therapies through experiences with patients asking questions that he could not answer. His own lack of knowledge on these topics prompted him to begin seeking information.

Irvin Boichuk is a qualified post-secondary instructor in British Columbia. He operates a publishing and training business, primarily developing educational materials.

Earle and Irvin have spent a great deal of time studying, researching and assembling the information contained in this publication. They have tried very hard to remain unbiased in the presentation of information.

Other people have provided input, effort and support in the development of this book.

Cheryl Boichuk was particularly vigilant against bias in the interpretation of the data.

Jane Price at the Nanaimo General Hospital has been invaluable. Our work would have been much more difficult without Jane as a source of data, general information and clinical study results.

Bonita McKay of *Today's Times* has steadfastly believed in this project. Her enthusiasm and drive have been inspirational.

It is our hope that knowledge will lead to better health through informed choices in therapy.

Introduction

Alternative therapies for all types of health problems have always been readily available. These therapies may be questionable, unorthodox, and unconventional, but they are used by many people who feel that they represent the "natural" approach to curing disease.

People seek help from dietary modifications, vitamins, exotic herbs, or chemical cures. They may even take expensive, unproven treatments in large clinics located in other countries. They seek these cures on the advice of friends, from information found in magazines and periodicals, or just on the basis of rumor.

Why do people seek unproven, questionable, and often dangerous cures? The reasons, while many and varied, naturally include the fear of death. Many people distrust the medical system and fear the conventional therapies that the system recommends. When those therapies offer no further hope, the terminal patient may try anything, including desperate measures, to survive. While most alternative therapies may not cause harm, some will have unpredictable side effects with serious, even fatal results. Such therapies, when used in conjunction with conventional therapies, may be especially dangerous.

For the oncologist, anticipating a five-year survival rate of 70% for a patient with cancer of the breast seems quite hopeful. From the victim's point of view, a 30% death rate is unacceptable.

For many cancer patients, the horror of the diagnosis is eclipsed by the horrors of the treatment. Radiation, surgery, and chemotherapy are not perfect cures without side effects. They may cause hair loss, nausea, vomiting, damage to blood-producing tissues, and many other problems. An alternative therapy may seem much less damaging and more natural, and it may even carry a false guarantee of success.

Prescribed, recognized remedies for arthritis also have side effects. These include dizziness, nausea, diarrhea, internal bleeding, and low white blood cell count. Arthritis sufferers may endure continuous, excruciating pain as well as severe impairment of mobility and independence. This also affects their self- esteem and pride. When the pain and discomfort become unbearable, and when conventional therapy does not seem to work effectively, patients may seek alternative therapies.

Alternative arthritis remedies have even higher risks. Although many of their side effects are dangerous, people still use alternatives, assuming that the medical profession is only out to "make a buck" on the recognized therapies and drugs while hiding the true cures behind precautionary statements.

It is estimated that the money spent annually by North Americans for unorthodox cures exceeds ten billion dollars.

Generally, over half of the cancer patients surveyed used some form of treatment other than the conventional medical therapy. Surveys reveal that the use of cancer "cures" increases with income and education. The physician plays a key role in encouraging or preventing the use of alternative methods by educating the patient about the hazards of unproven cures.

Estimates put the number of rheumatoid arthritis sufferers in Canada at more than 250,000. Every year they spend over two billion dollars on questionable remedies. In contrast, over twenty million dollars are donated to legitimate arthritis research.

Clearly, some natural alternative therapies have a beneficial effect on illness and the prevention of disease. The most effective preventive therapies include proper diet, standard medical practice, and carefully chosen alternatives. Unfortunately, it is difficult to locate concise, useful information that a physician or a patient can access readily with full understanding.

It is not the goal of this publication to be judgemental. Its purpose is to present as much factual material as possible to the physician and the patient considering an alternate therapy.

Chapter 1

ALTERNATIVES

15 / The Question of Alternatives
16 / The Scientific Method
18 / Product Regulations
21 / The Long List of Choices

ALTERNATIVES

The Question of Alternatives

Alternative therapies include any therapy that is not recognized by the medical associations or by the health organizations of any province, state or country. The dispute over whether or not the government has the right to determine what is recognized and what is not recognized as a medical treatment continues.

The Food and Drug Administration was established to protect us from unknown and dangerous chemicals, plants, and general foodstuffs. In the case of drugs, exhaustive testing ensures that the function of the drug is as stated and that all possible side effects are documented.

Most alternative therapies originate in religion or folklore, or through legends passed down by previous generations. Alternative medicines, therapies, and "cures" are options that most people will choose at some point in their lives. These alternatives will vary from dietary supplements and herbal teas to elaborate and potentially dangerous therapies.

The regulation of drugs and therapies has always annoyed the alternative medicine community. As Dr. Julian Whitaker states in an advertisement for his periodical *Health and Wellness Today*, " . . . the Food and Drug Administration has actually made it a crime for vitamin makers and health food stores to tell you about these amazing new therapies . . . when they've tried, FDA storm troopers have broken down their doors, confiscated their products and put them out of business."

The Scientific Method

Why are some therapies and drugs "recognized" while others are not? The answer is straightforward. New or questionable remedies can be placed in three basic categories:

- unknown
- experimental
- disproven

Unknown remedies are those which are new and have never been used before. These remedies must be tested and studied to determine if they will be accepted. Unfortunately, the high cost of continuous testing does not permit every remedy to undergo extensive study.

Experimental remedies are those that have potential for being effective and are undergoing testing to determine if they will fulfill the claims that have been made for their performance.

Disproven remedies are those which after extensive testing are found to be unsafe, ineffective, or fraudulent.

How do remedies become "recognized"? For example, suppose doctors or scientists discover a new use for a drug. To have its use considered for recognition by the

Food and Drug Administration, they would have to follow an established scientific method to prove the remedy. This system works this way:

Scientists test the drug, recording in detail the process used, including all active and non-active ingredients.

The drug is tested in an experimental group of patients, some of whom receive the drug while others receive a placebo. The term "placebo" is derived from Latin and means "I shall please." It is a harmless substance given to a patient in an experiment. In scientific terms, this type of experiment is called "a randomized double-blind trial against placebo." In the experiment, the patients do not know whether they are getting a drug or a harmless substance. In this way, there is no bias introduced into the test and the results will not be affected.

The more patients involved and the longer the time period of the test, the greater the accuracy of the results. Early testing is usually performed on animals rather than humans.

The test results are carefully recorded in a manner that will allow any other scientist to run the same experiment. This permits a wider study to determine if the result of the original test matches other tests. These test results are normally published in scientific or medical journals. During this testing period, the side effects of the drugs are determined, and the drug can be modified (if possible) to eliminate side effects or undesirable results.

When the results of the testing prove that the drug is safe for use with humans, tests are often performed on groups of human patients to further establish the results.

Following extensive testing, if the drug is proven to be effective and safe, it is accepted by the government agency responsible for safeguarding medication and is listed as an acceptable remedy.

Most alternative therapies or medications bypass the scientific process and are marketed directly to the consumer. Without any testing at all, these remedies cannot be considered effective or safe for use.

During scientific testing, it is not uncommon for up to 30% of the placebo group to show an improvement in symptoms. This improvement is often temporary, and it is directly related to mental attitude. The drug must not simply match the improvement of the placebo group; it must show significantly better results over a long period of time to be acceptable as a treatment.

With some ailments, such as arthritis, a patient often experiences a remission at about the same time that an alternate therapy is first applied. Remission does not mean cure, and the symptoms may return.

Product Regulations

Over-the-counter products that have not undergone any testing must still be regulated. These are considered homeopathic products and are still governed by the Food and Drugs Act. All products must carry a Drug Identification Number (DIN).

To qualify for a DIN, the product must be non-toxic, and it must be labelled according to certain regulations. These regulations require the manufacturer to state that the product is to be used only as directed by a physician or homeopathic practitioner. In addition, the label or any advertising relating to the product cannot claim any therapeutic activity or state any specific "cures" that will be achieved by using the product.

The problem with the regulation is that there is no legal definition for a "homeopathic practitioner." In Canada, anyone can practise homeopathy. Since homeopathic remedies are basically non-toxic and free from side effects, they are relatively harmless. In the United States, homeopathy is considered the practice of medicine, and only licensed health professionals are permitted to prescribe homeopathic medications. Despite the legalities of the systems, it is estimated that there are thousands of unskilled homeopaths practising medicine.

Unfortunately, many who accept this form of therapy also tend to abandon traditional medical care. This could obviously have a severe effect on a patient with a serious medical condition.

In the absence of adequate legislation, pharmacists have been offered guidelines by their associations to help in the distribution of homeopathic products. These guidelines state that

- pharmacies which offer these products should have a pharmacist with a knowledge of homeopathic remedies available for consultation;

- space should be available for consultation with patients;

- the same attention should be given to dispensing homeopathic medicines as is given prescription medication;

- pharmacies should maintain a good supply of information books regarding homeopathic substances and therapies; and that

- pharmacists should be aware of the possibilities of

hypersensitive reactions or aggravation of symptoms as a result of homeopathic preparations.

Alternative drugs and therapies are not ignored by science or the medical community. Many different alternatives have been tested and accepted as safe after extensive experimentation and documentation. Following a dramatic increase in the requests for DINs in the 1980s, the government issued proposals to modify the licensing system for these products. The concern was that many of the products were outside the realm of homeopathy and that the public might be misled as to their effectiveness or safety. These new proposals, issued in 1990, state that:

- the ingredient or ingredients must be listed in *Homeopathis Pharmacopoeia of the United States* or the *Pharmacopée Française;*
- the label will carry the identification "HM" rather than "DIN";
- the label cannot state any therapeutic claims; and
- the label must state that the effectiveness of the remedy in treating any disease has not been demonstrated by scientific method.

To date, the issue has not been resolved. In fact, there is question as to whether the products should be issued any number at all or if they should be regulated under completely different guidelines.

Currently, a vast variety of homeopathic remedies are available. These can be purchased in a number of pharmacies or by direct order from various companies. These remedies range from hair tonics to shark cartilage. They invariably contain some unknown, protected-by-copyright ingredient. Cures and remedies without DINs, varying from exotic herbal teas to energy pills, can be found in any health food store. The hazard of these remedies is that the user does not know what their active ingredients are or what effect they will have on the body.

The Long List of Choices

The list of alternative medicines and remedies is almost endless. Each alternate provides claims of effectiveness and extensive histories, some documented, others unsupported. While each is attractive for its application, remember that they are all unproven. We have tried to categorize the alternatives described in this book by the following:

- therapies that occur in clinics
- remedies involving specific chemicals
- therapies utilizing diets and vitamins
- remedies using herbs, plants, and other natural ingredients
- therapies involving religion, non-ingested items, and miscellaneous remedies

Clinic therapies are relatively straightforward. They occur in a specific location, are administered by a "specialist," and usually have a particular audience. For example, you would have to go to the Immunology Research Center in the Bahamas to get immunoaugmentative therapy for cancer.

Remedies with chemicals involve specific chemicals discovered or created for medicinal use. For example, dimethyl sulfoxide is often used in the treatment of cancer.

Therapies using vitamins and diets become somewhat confusing, since there are so many variations on diet. We have examined the macrobiotic diet in detail because of its popularity. This section also discusses herbal remedies, which include teas, creams, and broths.

The final category is very broad, since it involves a number of therapies that stretch beyond the realms of mind, religion, and attitude.

Some of the therapies that we could not place include the following:

INDUCTOSCOPES

These are electrical devices that will bombard you with magnetic waves to "cure" arthritis, cancer, or other ailments. Extended exposure to electromagnetism is currently under study as a cause of cancer.

COPPER BRACELETS

They cause no harm (unless you are allergic to copper). They have absolutely no effect, unless you abandon your regular, prescribed treatment plans, in which case your symptoms will get worse.

SOLARAMA BOARDS

These are supposed to realign your electrons into their proper position to cure your ailments. There is no evidence that they work as described by the manufacturer.

WD40

This is a lubricating product made from petroleum distillates. It is flammable and can cause respiratory disease, skin disease, and general allergic reaction. It will not cure arthritis or alleviate joint discomfort.

RADON

Radon is the radioactive gaseous by-product which occurs when radium atomically disintegrates. It has been reported to cure arthritis and cancer as well as a host of other ailments. Radon is a health hazard.

SNAKE VENOMS

Reputed to be valuable in the treatment of arthritis. There is no proof that they have any effect. They have been used by native healers to reduce swelling and pain; they do have minor anti-inflammatory properties. Use can cause extreme side effects and the possibility of life-threatening allergic reaction.

SNAKE CAPSULES

These contain the dried meat of rattlesnakes. They are claimed to be effective in the cure of arthritis. Some people who took these capsules developed salmonella food poisoning and discovered that their arthritic symptoms were also aggravated.

PECTIN

This product (commercially known as Certo) is used for making jams and jellies. Clinical tests following reports of effectiveness in treating arthritis have shown them to be false.

MUSSEL EXTRACT

Reported to have anti-inflammatory properties. Independent laboratory studies have not been able to produce any positive results.

FISH OILS

These may provide marginal results for persons suffering from rheumatoid arthritis. There is some possibility that the fatty acids synthesized from fish oils can inhibit some inflammatory chemicals in the body. There is no proof that they will provide any relief. Megadoses of cod-liver oil can cause vitamin D toxicity.

The list of possible remedies and therapies is endless. Many of them began as rumors and expanded with time and telling until they become "magic cures." Unfortunately, people tend to abandon a doctor's prescribed treatment and change their life-style and diet without even understanding what they are putting into their bodies—often with tragic consequences.

Galen (A.D. 130 to 201), the physician to the Roman Imperial Court and one of the founders of modern medicine, was quoted as saying "All who drink of this remedy are cured, except those who die. Thus it is effective for all but the incurable."

When you choose an alternate therapy, always consult with your physician. Even though doctors are constrained by the boundaries of science and medicine, they are still ultimately qualified to assist you in determining if an alternate therapy will help you or cause greater problems to your health. Additional information is available from a number of national resources, including the arthritis and cancer societies. You can also contact the Health Protection Branch, Department of Health and Welfare, at Tunney's Pasture, Ottawa, Ontario, K1A 0L2.

Chapter 2

CLINIC THERAPIES

27 / Antineoplastins
29 / Chacon Cancer Cure
31 / Gerson Therapy
36 / Greek Cure
38 / Immunoaugmentative Therapy
41 / Mexican Arthritis Treatments
43 / Psychic Surgery
47 / Simonton Method

CLINIC THERAPIES

Antineoplastins

Antineoplastins are the discovery of Stanislaw R. Burzynski, M.D. of the Burzynski Research Institute in Houston Texas. Burzynski was educated in Poland and is licensed to practise medicine in Texas. He and his associates have been working on antineoplastins as a new treatment for cancer since 1967.

Antineoplastins are described as substances which are produced by the living organism and which protect it against development of neoplastic tumor or growth but do not significantly inhibit the growth of normal tissues.

In 1982, antineoplastin treatment cost $180 per day. These treatments lasted from six weeks to a year and the total cost was about $5000 per month. Travel costs and any additional costs were not included. A deposit of $5000 was required.

CLAIMS FOR (UNVERIFIED)

According to Burzynski, antineoplastins act as "reverse oncogenes" (oncogenes are cancer-causing substances) which change malignant (cancerous) tissue back into normal tissue. Oncogenes are described as polypeptides derived from urine. Burzynski's theory is that a deficiency of antineoplastins in the body creates cancer, while treatment with them reverses cancer.

Burzynski claims that he has treated twenty-one patients who had advanced cancers such as breast, bladder, colon, and blood. Following treatment, 86% of the patients showed some clinical improvement without any evidence of significant toxicity and with minimal side effects.

CLAIMS AGAINST

Burzynski refuses to use the accepted scientific method of testing his products on animals. His claim is that since the drug is an extract from human urine, it will only work in humans and will have no effect on animals.

This biological substance is claimed to have dramatic anticancer activity. However, the compound is complex and has never been reproduced.

There are no firm supporting clinical reports, and the substance has not been made available for impartial testing and evaluation. The burden of proof remains with Dr. Burzynski to supply more convincing evidence.

To determine the facts about antineoplastins, the Ontario government sent two Toronto specialists to Burzynski's clinic. They reviewed twenty of the purported cases and determined that there was no evidence proving that anyone had benefited from treatment with antineoplastins. Three of four patients who Burzynski claimed had achieved complete remissions had died of recurrences. The fourth patient had undergone surgery, which was believed to be curative, for bladder cancer.

Careful surveillance of medical literature has revealed no additional reports of clinical trials.

The American Cancer Society does not recognize treatment with antineoplastins as an approved cancer therapy. The ACS has warned cancer patients against such treatment.[1]

According to *The Vancouver Sun*, a Port Alberni, British Columbia resident, Wayne Ingham, died in a Vancouver hospital after being treated with Burzynski's antineoplastins. When Ingham and his parents first returned to Port Alberni with a month's supply of medication they were very optimistic that the treatments had helped in curing his disease. After Ingham died, his parents said they had a renewed respect for Canadian medical treatment and ethics.[2]

Nine of eleven Cancer Control Agency of B.C. (CCABC) patients who were treated with antineoplastins died without receiving any therapeutic effect from the drugs. One other patient, who received curative treatment at CCABC went into remission. The last patient, Dr. Burzynski's "best case," responded extremely well to radiation therapy; however such a response was not unheard of and could not be credited to antineoplastins.[3]

Two Ontario patients who were treated in Texas developed septicemia, which is an infection of the bloodstream. One of them subsequently died. Stephanie Kusan, another Ontario patient, paid $75,000 for unsuccessful treatments by Dr. Burzynski.[4]

Chacon Cancer Cure

The Chacon Cancer Society was founded by Fernando Chacon Mejias of Cordoba, Spain. He claims that the society is working to provide solutions to the problems of cancer, rheumatism, non-bacterial rheumatic fever, Parkinson's disease, and an extensive range of other diseases. In the early 1970s the Chacon Cancer Society applied for patents in several countries for a process for preparing a vaccine against cancer and other similar diseases.

CLAIMS FOR (UNVERIFIED)

Mejias' diagnosis and treatment are based on his discovery of the third basic form of life. He claims that the first two forms are bacteria and viruses and that the third is a living enzyme. Such enzymes may either combine with genes or exist freely. If they combine with genes, they will form cancer, otherwise they will cause chronic, non-malignant disease such as arthritis.

Testing is based on his theory that many strains of bacteria will produce antigens when they react to a patient's antibodies which have been strengthened with living enzymes. He developed a universal test using a bacterial extract which will separate when heated, thus proving the existence of the enzymes.

CLAIMS AGAINST

The Cancer Control Agency of British Columbia cautions that any treatment that has no established foundation in fact is unlikely to be of any real value. The Chacon Cancer Cure is similar to most cancer "cures" in that it links a testing procedure to a treatment which uses natural procedures and gives the patient a panacea which claims to be effective for all types of cancer, including any chronic, non-malignant disease. For this cure, there have been no clinical studies, toxicity tests, efficacy tests or independent statements from any source indicating that there is any validity to the claims of remission or outright cure. No laboratory tests have been performed on either animals or humans to substantiate the claims.[5]

The testing process used to prove the existence of the enzymes and the effects of treatment was quite popular at the turn of the century. It was quite common before modern biochemistry discovered more accurate and efficient methods of testing.

Gerson Therapy

Dr. Max Gerson was born in Wongrowitz, Germany in 1881. He developed a low-salt diet with a high level of fresh fruit and vegetables that helped to control his migraine headaches. He applied his diet to his tuberculosis patients and observed that they improved. He documented his application of his diet in a book titled *A Cancer Therapy: Results of Fifty Cases*.

His proponents continue to practise his therapy in Tijuana, Mexico. His cancer therapy is considered unacceptable by the United States medical establishment.

The therapy consists of a low-sodium, high-potassium, poison-free diet in conjunction with coffee enemas. Enemas originated with fifth-century healers who claimed that inducing continuous bowel movements removed "corrupt humors" from the body. This became known as "purging." The concept of purging with enemas continued as a regular practice through the nineteenth century.

The Gerson therapists maintain that an unpoisoned body has special reserves that can recognize and destroy cancer. They define cancer as a degenerative disease that develops when oxidative energy normally occurring in the liver is converted to fermentative energy by poisons from processed food. They believe that the body can be cleansed of all toxins by coffee enemas and maintained in that condition by a specific diet.

The diet consists of drinking juices made from calf liver and raw fruits and vegetables grown without the use of any chemicals, pesticides, herbicides, fungicides or fertilizers. The juice must also be prepared without chemicals, sugar, starch, salt or preservatives. The diet is supplemented with megadoses of vitamins, Laetrile, minerals and oxygenators. Additions to the diet may include acid pepsin, potassium, and extracts of thyroid.

Virtually no other fluids are permitted, including alcohol, tea or coffee. The coffee forms an important part of the treatment, but only in the form of enemas applied every four hours. Patients may have soap and water enemas on alternate days.

According to the information on the Word Wide Web (1995), cost for the Gerson treatment at the clinic in Mexico is approximately $4500 U.S. per week, not including extras such as tests, transportation, day charges for patients and their companions, and Mexican taxes. The clinic recommends six weeks of therapy.

CLAIMS FOR (UNVERIFIED)

According to Gerson, in normal cell operation, the aerobic energy metabolism is maintained by oxygen and the oxidizing enzymes. If processed foods are introduced to the system, the cells are poisoned by the toxins and begin to use fermentation for energy production. Because this type of energy production is inferior, the cells become malignant. The potassium in the cells becomes inactive and the sodium minerals become negatively ionized.

By using coffee enemas, the bile duct becomes dilated, stimulates bile production and activates the neutralization of free radicals in the blood and tissues of the body. This process removes the toxins from the body through the gall bladder and intestine as bile salts to the colon to be excreted. The enema passes through the wall of the bowel to dilute toxins passing into the liver. The toxins are flushed down the intestine along with metabolites from the tumor.

The coffee in the enema stimulates bile production and formation because of two ingredients found in coffee: kahweol and cafestol.

Diet is important in maintaining a poison-free system and for stimulating the energy metabolism in the cells. This diet of juices restores normal function to poison-damaged organs. The enzymes in the juice replace the enzymes in the vital organs, thus restoring them to their proper condition. The essential organs in the body can then produce an allergic inflammatory reaction that will selectively kill cancer cells.

CLAIMS AGAINST

The amount of information available on the causes, progression, and initiation of cancer since Gerson promoted this therapy is vast. Studies as early as 1961 determined that there is no relationship between cell malignancy and fermentative energy production. Tumor cells will grow quite rapidly in tissue where an adequate supply of oxygen exists. The generation of energy from tumors comes from the oxidative metabolism of fats and carbohydrates, not from fermentation. There is no evidence that tumors poison the enzyme system.

Using bile to remove large quantities of poison from the system would be extremely inefficient, since more than 95% of the bile in the small intestine returns to the portal circulation and the liver before reaching the colon. This means that the poisons would actually be reabsorbed into the bloodstream and recirculated throughout the body. There are orally administered drugs that will bind with the poisons while they are still in the intestine and prevent them from returning with the bile.

Bile salts are required in the body to absorb fat-soluble vitamins and calcium. They regulate the synthesis of cholesterol and aid in the digestion of dietary fat. Enema flushing over a short period of time will remove very few bile salts. Flushing over long periods of time will remove significant amounts of bile salts. This removal will cause a number of nutritional problems due to the inability of the body to absorb fat, fat-soluble vitamins, and calcium.

Although most of the side effects of continuous purging are not reported by the clinics that perform these functions, some have been reported and documented. Coffee enemas have caused death by hyponatremia and dehydration. There was an outbreak of sepsis (infection of the blood from bacterial micro-organisms) in a Mexican clinic, and heavy fecal contamination of the apparatus caused amebic dysentery among patients receiving colon irrigation.

The coffee beans used to make the enemas at the clinic are roasted and ground. Roasting coffee beans destroys the kahweol and cafestol, thus reducing their stimulating activity.

There has never been any experimental evidence presented which shows that coffee enemas will stimulate bile production.

The ability of the body to absorb enzymes is extremely low. Enzymes that are absorbed are normally recognized by the body as foreign and are captured and destroyed by the immune system. Because they are foreign enzymes, they are dismantled into amino acids in the gastrointestinal tract. If the enzyme could survive and enter the system, it would have to locate the damaged organ, enter the cells of that organ, and insert itself into the appropriate intracellular structure. The introduction of foreign enzymes into the circulation system of a human could cause a dangerous immune response.

Clinical trials indicate that allergic inflammatory reaction actually causes death or injury to normal cells. Fat metabolism in the cell is reduced, and the cell reverts to fermentation as the oxidative energy production falls. This induces septic shock, hemorrhagic necrosis, and organ damage. The effects and changes that occur during this process are basically the same as the effects identified as causing the cancer originally. Blood tests of patients using Gerson therapy have never shown an increase in natural killer cells, immune response mediators, or cytotoxic T-cells.

In clinical tests, the placebo used with the Gerson diet has been equally effective in treating cancer.

Greek Cure

The Greek Cure for Cancer is associated with Greek physician Hariton Alivizatos, M.D. Dr. Alivizatos' specialty is in microbiology, and he is accredited by the Athens Medical Society.

At the time Dr. Alivizatos' clinic was operating, cost of the treatment was $50 for each blood test and $40 for each injection. Treatment normally consisted of about eighteen to twenty injections. Treatment took from one to three years. Costs for travel and accommodation were not included. The doctor insisted on payment by cash or traveller's checks.

Dr. Alivizatos has carefully guarded the secret of his medication. He is reported willing to sell the formula for seven million dollars.

CLAIMS FOR (UNVERIFIED)

Dr. Alivizatos claims to have developed a special blood test that can determine the type and location of a patient's cancer and rate severity on a scale from 0 to 10. He also claims to have a treatment to cure cancer. This treatment prevents the onset of cancer, dissolves tumors, and restores tissue to its normal healthy state.

The treatment is in the form of serum injections which strengthen the patient's immune system and help the fight to destroy cancer cells. These cancer cells are excreted through the patient's natural body waste as part of the natural function. At the same time, the serum helps the body rejuvenate those cells or parts of the body that are being destroyed by cancer.

Leukemia patients cannot be treated if they are taking morphine or methadone, as this will cause a reaction. Leukemia patients can be treated if the heaviest medication being taken is Percodan. Dr. Alivizatos claims to have a 99% cure rate.

CLAIMS AGAINST

A literature search by the American Cancer Society Medical Library found no publications that were relevant to Dr. Alivizatos' work. The ACS has twice requested documentation from Dr. Alivizatos, but he has not replied.

Dr. Alivizatos claims to have documentation from the past twenty-two years of six thousand Greek patients who were treated in his clinic. This is apparently on file with the Greek Commission of Drugs.

The ACS has also been unable to confirm that the Greek Minister of Health has the formula for the serum, that laboratories in Geneva are testing the serum, or that the serum even exists.

The American Cancer Society does not recognize Greek Cure as an approved cancer treatment. The ACS has strongly cautioned patients not to participate in such treatment.[6]

The Greek government closed Dr. Alivizatos' clinic after a sample of medicine was analyzed and shown to be nicotinic acid (niacin). An American doctor had posed as a patient and had shipped a sample back to an American laboratory.[7]

Immunoaugmentative Therapy

Immunoaugmentative therapy (IAT) is advocated by Lawrence Burton, Ph.D. Burton has a Ph.D. from New York University (1955). His doctoral dissertation was titled "Carcinogenic activity of larval donor extracts in *Drosophila*" (fruit flies). From 1955-57 he worked at the California Institute of Technology. From 1959 on he worked at the Hodgkin's Disease Research Laboratory, St. Vincent's Hospital, New York City.

In 1973, Burton formed The Immunology Research Foundation in Great Neck, N.Y. He moved the foundation to Freeport, Bermuda in 1977 because the U.S. Food and Drug Administration continued to refuse to grant permission for clinical trials of an immunological approach to the treatment of cancer.

A fee schedule from Dr. Burton's center lists the following:

- a fee of $350 payable at time of evaluation for a review of records and clinical laboratory work and immunocompetence testing
- a fee of $3000 payable upon acceptance for four weeks of therapy
- a fee of $450 per week for the fifth week and each week thereafter

Patients remain in treatment for a minimum of six to eight weeks. If they go home, they must return for a three- to five-day period after twelve to sixteen weeks. Transportation costs are not included.

It is estimated that over 1900 cancer patients travelled to Bermuda between 1977 and 1983 to receive immunoaugmentative therapy.

CLAIMS FOR (UNVERIFIED)

Lawrence Burton, Antonio Rottino, Frank Friedman, Robert Kassell and John Harris found natural substances that caused approximately 50% remissions of leukemia in mice.

The Immunology Research Center claims 50% response rates with humans in a wide variety of tumors and several diseases treatable by more conventional strategies. These include previously untreatable cancers such as:

- ovarian
- prostate
- small-cell histiocytic lymphoma
- acute leukemias

A pamphlet from the Immunology Research Center claims that since the therapy will reverse the progress of cancer and correct the immunological faults in animals, it will also do the same for humans with similar faults. The Center maintains that continued use of the treatment will correct faults in the immune system.[8]

Dr. Burton claims to have found certain factors in blood that have an anti-cancer effect. He also claims to have identified a "blocking" protein which inhibits the immune system. According to Burton, a developing tumor stimulates the body to produce tumor complement. Tumor complement in turn activates tumor antibody. However, the blocking protein interrupts this process. Therefore Dr. Burton's treatment includes a "deblocking" protein which neutralizes the blocking protein and allows the natural working of the immune system.[9]

CLAIMS AGAINST

Although statements by Dr. Burton roughly coincide with some prevailing immunological theories, no actual data has ever been offered to support the alleged relation to the product produced by the Immunology Research Center. The method of preparation is kept secret and only the Research Center can make the drug for distribution.

In 1978 the National Cancer Institute (NCI) of the U.S. Department of Health and Human Services stated that the clinic records were inadequate and could not be accurately evaluated. Dr. Burton would not reveal the composition of the treatment materials or the method for preparing them.

In 1984, the National Cancer Institute offered to screen Dr. Burton's materials to evaluate the antitumor properties of the treatment. They also suggested possible collaboration and approaches for evaluating his methods. However, Dr. Burton refused to reveal the composition and method of production of the drug, and the National Cancer Institute would not participate in human testing without knowing what they were testing.

The NCI tested samples of IAT reagents used in five patients and found all of them contaminated with bacteria (pseudomonas, corynebacterium, staphylococcus, bacillus, propionibacterium, and achromobacter species). Four of the samples contained hepatitis B surface antigen or anticore antibody or both. One of the patients actually contracted hepatitis.[10]

From March 1982 to March 1984, sixteen persons who had received treatment at the Center developed abscesses at injection sites. Organisms recovered from the abscesses included *Nocardia asteroides, Staphylococcus aureus, Escherichia coli* and an unidentified Actinomyces-like organism.

Organ transplant patients, who receive immuno-suppressive drugs, and cancer patients have a higher risk of infection. In 1985, two patients who attended the clinic provided samples of serum proteins to labs in Washington. All eighteen of these samples tested positive for HBsAg, and eight of the eighteen tested either positive or borderline for HTLV III (the virus associated with AIDS). The Center for Disease Control (CDC) consistently found viable HTLV III in one of the samples.[11]

In August 1985, newspapers reported the evidence of AIDS virus in IAT material. The Freeport clinic was closed and Burton announced that he was moving to Mexico. The Bahamas clinic has since reopened on the understanding that blood products will be tested for hepatitis antigen and evidence of AIDS virus before being used on patients.

It is reported that Burton's clinic was grossing at least $30 million a year before being closed.

Treatment continues in the absence of any evidence of therapeutic value or proof that the material even contains any active ingredient.

Mexican Arthritis Treatments

A number of clinics have been established in Mexico and in other Central American countries to cure inflammatory and rheumatoid arthritis as well as other joint disorders. Because of its easy access from the United States, Mexico is a preferred site.

These clinics provide diagnosis and treatment through the use of drugs which are not accepted as safe by food and drug administrations in North America.

CLAIMS FOR

Patients using these clinics have shown marked improvement in functional ability, mobility, and pain reduction or elimination. In some patients, weight gain has improved and, in general, the benefits of the treatment were substantial.

CLAIMS AGAINST

Most of the treatments administered by these clinics are not recognized as safe by the national food and drug administrations of many countries. In addition, the drugs administered are often misrepresented. The following table shows some of the declared treatments and their actual contents as determined by laboratory analysis.

Alleged treatment	Chemical analysis
indomethacin	diazepam
naproxen	generic steroids
tanderil	generic steroids
diazepam	diazepam
DMSO	phenylbutazone,
muscle relaxant	dyperone or
	generic steroids
	diazepam

The treatments are normally issued in yellow-, white-, or green-coloured capsules. Testing showed that almost all of the capsules contained generic steroids. While steroid treatment will provide almost instantaneous relief from arthritis and joint discomfort, the side effects of this type of treatment are extensive and life-threatening.

Some of the chemicals, such as dyperone, are used in veterinary medicine as analgesics and are not safe for human use because of the extreme side effects. All of the anti-inflammatories can cause peptic ulcers and kidney failure, and phenylbutazone can cause fatal bone marrow depression.

Steroid or cortisone medications have a long list of side effects. These include gastric ulcers (often with bleeding), destruction of joints, weight gain, fluid retention, heart failure, acne, and many others. Cortisone suppresses the inflammatory component of the immune system and masks the body's response to other diseases. The absence of symptoms (such as fever and pain) may result in serious disease going undetected until it is too late. Cortisone also activates latent tuberculosis and causes the disease to develop rapidly.

The side effects of cortisone therapy are always a concern to a physician prescribing these drugs. They become much more dangerous when neither the patient nor doctor are aware that they are being used.

One study of six patients who attended Mexican arthritis clinics found that the patients were not told what drugs they received or warned of the dangerous and possibly life-threatening side effects. Overall improvement of symptoms was short-lived and not able to be sustained with conventional therapy.[12]

Psychic Surgery

It is estimated that there are at least four hundred psychic surgeons in the Philippines. These surgeons claim that they can enter the body with their bare hands and remove tumors, blood clots and other organic material without the use of anesthetics. The surgery leaves no scars or pain, and many patients believe, at least for a time, that they have been cured.

Each large hotel in Manila has a resident psychic surgeon. The most famous of all psychics was the Reverend Tony Agpaoa. He created a special travel agency, Diplomat Tours, which took organized groups from Europe, North America, Japan, Australia, and New Zealand to the Philippines for healing sessions. He was not permitted to organize tours from the United States for legal reasons.

The cost of an organized tour from Edmonton to Manilla was about $1,533 in Canadian funds.

In 1967 Tony Agpaoa was indicted for fraud in the United States for psychic surgery. He forfeited a $25,000 bond, jumped bail, and returned to the Philippines. He is now deceased.

CLAIMS FOR (UNVERIFIED)
Psychic surgeons claim that they can cure many diseases including diabetes and cancer. The causes of disease include imbalances in the body, biofeedback, and mental consciousness. Healing the disease is of secondary importance.

Primary importance is given to bringing back a natural way of life to make people healthy again. The psychic surgeon guarantees that people will leave in a better physical and spiritual state, but he can't guarantee that they will be cured of their diseases.

Whether psychic surgery operations are legitimate is irrelevant to the surgeons. Dramatic operations give patients more confidence and faith in the healing and are no different nor more morally wrong than a western doctor prescribing a placebo.

Psychic surgeons claim that their patients heal themselves. Psychic surgery plants the seed that the patient's mind uses to complete the cure. A report recently made by the Yukon Medical Association notes that many individuals who underwent psychic surgery showed marked subjective improvement. However, all of these cases had poorly defined, nonspecific disorders such as headaches, abdominal pain, or back pain.

CLAIMS AGAINST

Psychic healers often remove objects such as pieces of tinfoil, coins, chicken feet, or other foreign objects during their operation. This is because the Filipinos believe that evil spirits put these objects into people to make them sick. When dealing with westerners, the healers imitate more orthodox medical operations so that they can convince their patients that they are legitimate.

The real danger of psychic surgery is not in the psychic surgeon's actions, but in sick people ignoring proper medical care in their search for a miracle. Most often, their return to recognized medical doctors and practices occurs too late.

The Philippine Medical Association (PMA) claims that psychic surgeons take advantage of the gullibility of people. It cannot prevent the practice or take legal action against it because there is no proof that any violations have taken place. Patients don't like to admit they have been made fools of, so they don't complain.

In the past two years, the Canadian Embassy in Manila has signed three death certificates for people who did not return alive from their miracle tours. According to the Cancer Control Agency of B.C., of more than twenty known cancer cases who went to Baguio from Vancouver, not one is still alive.

Donald and Carol Wright of Iowa, students and believers in ESP and magnetic surgery, travelled to the Philippines to study psychic surgery. They later testified before a U.S. Federal Trade Commission which was investigating travel agents who were promoting tours to the Philippines for psychic healing. The Wrights lost their faith in the treatment after they were taught by Philippine surgeon teachers how to shop for the right animal parts to make a "bullet." This bullet was composed of cotton and animal tissue or clots of animal blood; the Wrights were actually taught how to simulate its removal from the patient.[13]

The Province reported the case of Donald Douglas who travelled to the Philippines under the pretense of having a "bad heart." In fact, there was nothing wrong with him. His Philippine healer yanked a tumor the size of a peach pit out of Donald's body and immediately disposed of it before he could get a good look at it. Douglas said there was blood involved in the process, but that he was sure that it was animal or perhaps chicken blood. According to *The Province*, Gerry Galiau, a representative from the Philippine embassy in Ottawa, stated that his country believes that the healers are "shady" and estimates that they cheat people out of millions of dollars each year.[14]

Simonton Method

Dr. O. Carl Simonton is a medical doctor and a certified therapeutic radiologist. He is currently the Medical Director of the Cancer Counselling and Research Center in Azle, Texas.

The Simonton method consists of positive imaging by cancer patients in an effort to mobilize their ability to fight cancer.

In 1982 the fees for a ten-day session were $1,900 U.S. Transportation and living expenses were not included in this price.

CLAIMS FOR (UNVERIFIED)

Dr. Simonton claims that his technique approximately doubles survival time in most cancer patients.

Although the psychotherapeutic component of the therapy (relaxation and stress combat) is emphasized, advocates state that the approach has definite therapeutic effects against cancer and is much more than a relaxation technique.

The basic approach at the Cancer Counseling and Research Center is to use techniques in relaxation and mental imagery in cancer therapy. Patients are encouraged to imagine their body's immune cells destroying their cancer. This establishes a feeling of being in control of their lives and their disease. The staff at the Center emphasize that their methods are to be used in addition to orthodox cancer treatment; they do not advocate abandonment of standard medical therapy.

CLAIMS AGAINST

The division of Medical Oncology and the Management Committee of The Cancer Control Agency of B.C. (CCBAC) have reviewed the relevant publications from the Simontons, and as well have studied the report regarding their treatment prepared by the American Cancer Society (ACS) and offer the following comments:

• The Simontons have not evaluated their form of treatment in a scientific fashion.

• In 1981, the Simontons indicated to the American Cancer Society that a scientific evaluation was being done, but no such reports have appeared.

• The statistical method that the Simontons use to evaluate their therapy is simply not valid and would not allow one to draw any conclusions as to its usefulness.

An independent review of the Simontons by a group of psychiatrists and consultants in psychosomatic medicine for the American Cancer Society came to the following conclusions:

• There is no evidence indicating that the Simonton approach provides any therapeutic effect in patients with cancer.

• There is no evidence available that indicates that mental attitudes or degrees of stress influence the rate of progression or regression of malignant disease.

• Articles cited by the Simontons are highly selective, and they omit results of several studies which found no correlation between mental attitudes and progression of disease.

- Some patients may benefit psychologically from the feeling that they are in control of their disease; however when the disease progresses despite the use of the Simonton approach, patients may develop serious feelings of guilt and inadequacy and may develop a resulting severe depression.

- There is a definite risk that patients might abandon orthodox medical treatment even though they are discouraged from doing so by the staff at the Center.

- Patients using this approach on their own or receiving instruction from individuals not at the Simonton Clinic might substitute the method for standard medical therapy.

There is a difference between psychological and counselling techniques that are designed to relieve stress, combat anxiety, and encourage positive attitudes and those approaches that make claims for a specific anti-cancer action. "It is because it falls in this latter category that the Simonton method has to be classified as an unproved method of cancer treatment and not simply as a form of inducing psychological relaxation."[15]

The American Cancer Society, after studying all literature and documentation, does not have evidence that treatment with O. Carl Simonton's psychotherapy method results in any benefit in the treatment of cancer in human beings.

Chapter 3

CHEMICAL THERAPIES

53 / Dimethyl Sulfoxide
55 / Hydrazine Sulfate
58 / Laetrile
63 / Palcossio 55
63 / Pannon
64 / Pharmacological Therapies
66 / Tetracycline

CHEMICAL THERAPIES

Dimethyl Sulfoxide

Dimethyl sulfoxide is also known as DMSO. DMSO has been used as an industrial solvent since the 1940s. It is also a by-product of the paper industry. DMSO can pass through skin and travel into body tissue.

In the 1970s, British scientists tested DMSO on animals and discovered that it would protect tissue and cells from damage due to freezing. There was also some evidence that it would protect against radiation damage to cells and tissue.

DMSO first received publicity when a U.S. governor stated that he had used a veterinary form of DMSO to relieve the pain that his wife suffered as a result of terminal bone cancer.

Stanley Jacobs M.D., a professor of surgery at Oregon Health Science University, was one of the first to experiment with DMSO in treating different medical conditions. He believed that it might become a vehicle for administering cancer drugs into tumors, since it could penetrate the skin and tissues with relative ease.

The treatment for cancer at the Degenerative Disease Medical Center takes approximately four weeks. The estimated cost for treatment alone is approximately $4,000. This does not include any other expenses, such as travel and accommodations.

CLAIMS FOR (UNVERIFIED)

DMSO is used in the Degenerative Disease Medical Center in Las Vegas. This center is owned and administered by Mrs. Mildred Miller, who is also the editor of *Preventive Health News*. This is a monthly magazine that promotes DMSO as a treatment for different afflictions which include arthritis, mental illness, emphysema, and cancer.

Over a two-year period, the Center claimed to have treated thirty patients with advanced brain tumors. The patients received intravenous and oral Laetrile, DMSO, and metabolic therapy. This type of therapy uses vitamins, enzymes, and coffee retention enemas. The Center claimed that study of those treatments indicated that the thirty patients are in various stages of regression as follows:

- Six patients have had a reduction in the size of the brain tumor or had total remission (based on the results of brain scan testing).
- Two patients have had partial regression (based on the results of brain scan testing).
- Two have had prolongation of life.

The description of the procedure maintains that the cancer patient's immune system forms a protective shell around the cancer cell. DMSO can penetrate the shell and carry other medication directly to the cancerous cell.

Procaine hydrochloride is also given intravenously to cancer patients who receive the DMSO treatment, because it is believed that it increases the speed of pain relief.

Life Extension Products states that DMSO has been used successfully in conjunction with chemotherapy and has all of the desirable qualities of an effective cancer drug. The company claims that DMSO is possibly the most effective anti-cancer agent available.

CLAIMS AGAINST

The American Cancer Society does not endorse treatment with DMSO either alone or in conjunction with Laetrile or procaine hydrochloride. The Society strongly warns cancer patients against treatment with DMSO. Conventional medicine stopped using DMSO in the 1960s because of changes in the eyes of lab animals who were given the chemical.[1]

DMSO does take other products with it as it moves through the body tissues. As a result, the use of DMSO could prove fatal, particularly to a person who is already weakened by cancer. If used as a retention enema, DMSO could carry bacterial toxins from the rectum through the intestinal wall and into the bloodstream. This would result in a life-threatening situation.[2]

Hydrazine Sulfate

Hydrazine sulfate is also known as hydrazinium sulfate and hydra-zonium sulfate ($H_6N_2O_4S$). It is used

- for the gravimetric estimation of nickel, cobalt, and cadmium;
- for the refining of rare metals;

- as an antioxidant in solder flux for light metals;
- as a reducing agent in the processing of minerals;
- for separating polonium from tellurium;
- in tests for blood;
- for destroying fungi and molds; and
- in the preparation of hydrazine hydrate.

It was also used in rocket fuel during World War II.

CLAIMS FOR (UNVERIFIED)

Dr. J. Gold's tests with hydrazine sulfate led him to conclude that the chemical, a gluconeogenic blocking agent, interrupts the process of tumor growth at the expense of the host's energy. It is therefore beneficial for patients with cancer cachexia.[3] (Cachexia is weight loss, weakness, and debility.)

According to Gold, patients who received hydrazine sulfate had subjective improvement and their tumors regressed.[4]

CLAIMS AGAINST

Other researchers could not document or reproduce Dr. Gold's lab results.[5]

The Memorial Sloan-Kettering Cancer Center performed studies to evaluate the therapeutic value of hydrazine sulfate in treating humans. These tests resulted in the following conclusions:

- Significant subjective improvements or objective antitumor responses were not observed in any of twenty-nine patients treated with hydrazine sulfate.
- Four patients had briefly improved appetites without weight gain.

- One patient experienced a transitory decrease in bone pain without parallel improvement in the roentgenograms (x-rays) of the bones but with continuing elevations of the serum acid phosphatase (an enzyme produced by prostate cancer).

- The rate of accumulation of ascites decreased in one patient but prior paracenteses (draining of fluid from the abdominal cavity) had been performed.[6]

Researchers used hydrazine sulfate on live rats and mice which had tumors to study the chemical's effect on the gluconeogenesis (production of glucose) in their livers and kidneys. Although intensity of gluconeogenesis changed, decreasing in the liver and increasing in the kidneys, blood glucose content remained constant. From the data obtained, researchers were unable to support Dr. Gold's hypothesis.[7]

The following symptoms have been reported following the use of hydrazine sulfate for treatment:

- nausea
- vomiting
- anorexia
- abnormal sensations affecting both upper and lower extremities
- impaired fine motor functions
- confusion
- minor decrease in fasting blood sugar
- elevation in the serum activity of alkaline phosphatase
- elevation in the serum concentration of bilirubin
- abnormal electromyograms

- excitement
- lethargy
- convulsions
- hypotension (abnormally low blood pressure)
- arrhythmia (irregular heart beat)
- fatty changes in the liver
- hypoglycemia
- weight loss
- terminal changes in SGOT activity

Even very low doses of hydrazine sulfate were enough to act as carcinogens (cancer-causing substances) in the lungs of laboratory mice.[8]

Experiments performed in Switzerland showed that both hydrazine and methyl hydrazine produced lung tumors in mice.[9]

When hydrazine sulfate was studied as a tumor-causing agent in both male and female virgin mice, it induced lung tumors in 84% of the males and in 72% of the females. It also induced lung tumors in the F1 generation which was exposed during gestation, during lactation and post-weaning.[10]

Laetrile

The terms "Laetrile" and "amygdalin" are often used interchangeably. Although they are not chemically identical, they both belong to a family of compounds called cyanogenic glycosides.

These chemicals are found in the seeds of bitter almonds, peaches, and apricots. When extracted from oil of bitter almonds, the yield is 2 units of glucose, 1 unit of benzaldehyde and 1 unit of hydrogen cyanide.

Amygdalin was first discovered by Dioscorides of Anazarbos two thousand years ago. It was rediscovered in 1920 by a California physician, Ernest Krebs. He was experimenting with flavorings for bootleg whiskey. His son, Dr. Ernest Krebs, Jr., claimed in 1952 to have purified amygdalin, and he named it "Laetrile." It is usually administered in the form of bitter almonds.

CLAIMS FOR (UNVERIFIED)
Laetrile advocates advance two theories:

1. Cyanide release theory
Malignant tumors contain beta-glucosidase, an enzyme which causes Laetrile to release enough hydrogen cyanide to destroy cancerous tissue.[11]

2. Vitamin deficiency theory
Cancer is caused by vitamin deficiency, and Laetrile is actually a missing vitamin named B_{17}.[12]

CLAIMS AGAINST
None of the reputable scientific journals report any research that supports either of these two theories.[13]

1. Cyanide release theory
Dr. Charles G. Moertel described a clinical trial involving 178 patients. Patients were selected who had histologically (microscopically) proven cancer for which no standard treatment was known to be curative or to extend life expectancy. All patients had not had surgery, radiation therapy, or chemotherapy for one month. The amygdalin

used for treatment was prepared from apricot pits and supplied by the Pharmaceutical Resources Branch of the National Cancer Institute.

The routes, dosage and schedule of administration were chosen to be representative of current Laetrile practice.

Patients were also placed on a diet identical to the one recommended by most Laetrile practitioners.

Patients selected were in good general condition, were ambulatory (able to walk about), and able to maintain good nutrition. Patients who were disabled and bedridden were ineligible for the study.

In addition, eligible patients had either a tumor that could be measured in two dimensions or a clearly measurable liver enlargement due to cancer. Lesions had to be 5 cm in diameter to be acceptable for the study.[14]

After ten weeks of treatment, of 171 fully documented patients, only one patient met the criteria for partial response. This patient had changed physicians during the study and it is possible that the apparent response was actually a reflection of the expected variation inherent in two investigators assessing a tumor nodule. The patient died thirty-seven weeks after the start of therapy.

Fifty-four percent of the patients had measurable progression of malignant disease at the termination of their course of treatment. Seventy-nine percent of the patients had progression by two months. Ninety-one percent of the patients had progression by three months. All patients had progression by seven months.

Of the 178 patients entered before May 1981, 152 had died as of January 1982. The median survival time of these patients was 4.8 months.

Of the major tumor groups studied, median survival times were five months for lung cancer patients, four months for breast cancer patients, and three months for melanoma (skin cancer) patients. These results appeared consistent with survival times for patients receiving placebos or no treatment at all. More than half the patients had measurably larger tumors when they stopped receiving amygdalin therapy, and over 90% of them had progression by three months.[15]

2. Vitamin deficiency theory

Vitamins are required in small amounts for over-all health. They are not energy sources or sources of structural tissue; rather they promote vital physiological processes. Except for vitamin D, vitamins cannot synthesized by the cells. Certain diseases result from a deficiency in specific vitamins. These diseases are prevented or cured with those specific vitamins.[16]

In contrast, Laetrile is not required by the human body; it has not been shown to be associated with any vital physiological process. No disease has been linked to a deficiency in Laetrile.[17]

Some of the patients in Moertel's study had symptoms of toxicity. These symptoms disappeared when oral amygdalin was stopped. Some (but not all) of the patients had levels of blood cyanide high enough to be lethal to animals.[18]

Some sources of drug products have no enforced standards of quality or purity. Amygdalin imported from a major Mexican manufacturer, for instance, has frequently been found to be contaminated with bacteria.[19]

Amygdalin is non-toxic when injected, unless it is combined with a source of beta-glucosidase. However,

61

amygdalin taken orally is toxic, probably because beta-glucosidase is present in the small intestine.[20]

Amygdalin can be lethal if it is eaten along with a plant material containing beta-glucosidase.[21]

There are many reported cases in the literature of poisoning resulting from eating plant material containing both cyanogenic glycosides and beta-glucosidase. Ground apricot meal was the cause of several cases reported in California.[22]

Two reported deaths, one of a child, the other of a seventeen-year-old girl, occurred as a result of ingesting amygdalin preparations which were supposed to treat cancer.[23]

Researchers suspect that continued ingestion of cyanogenic glycoside in plant material causes tropical amblyopia and other obscure neurological disorders.[24]

Researchers suspect Laetrile may be a carcinogen (cancer-causing substance); they have observed genetic changes as determined by the Ames salmonella lyphimurium test.[25]

According to *The Los Angeles Times,* a breast-cancer patient who took massive doses of Laetrile subsequently died of cyanide poisoning.[26]

Another report, in *The Vancouver Sun,* stated that Chicago researchers had administered increasing doses of Laetrile to rats with tumors in order to determine the effects of the drug. According to their test results, increasing doses led to increases in tumor size and to eventual death from cyanide poisoning.[27]

The Richardson Center in Reno, Nevada requires a $2000 deposit on the first visit and charges up to $3000 per month for the first four months.[28]

Travel and room-and-board costs are not included. One Laetrile promoter was reported to have made a profit of $150,000 to $200,000 a month.[29]

Palcossio 55

Dr. M. A. Palencia, of Atlantis University in Barranguilla, Colombia, has created a chemical extracted from buzzard gastric juices. This chemical is called Palcossio 55. Dr. Palencia claims that it acts as an anticancer agent.

Atlantis University is not listed in the standard directory, *World of Learning*, although many other universities in Colombia are listed.

The National Cancer Institute was unable to supply any information on Palcossio 55 because the substance has not been submitted to be screened for antitumor activity. Similarly, the MEDLINE, TOXLINE, and CANCERLINE of the National Library of Medicine were also unable to provide any information on the substance.[30]

Pannon

Pannon is made by a small development-stage company in Bloomfield, N.J. called Alfacell. Pannon's composition is a well-guarded secret. The only description of the compound is that it is derived from living animal donor tissue. Pannon was formerly known as NSTT (Non-Specific Tumor Toxic) agent.

In April 1985, KCTS 9 in Seattle aired a program about Pannon as an anticancer agent. As a result, the Cancer Control Agency of British Columbia Library received many requests for information about the treatment. The library contacted KCTS, but the station was unable to identify the program from the descriptions given by the viewers. The library has been unable to obtain any further information about this anticancer agent.[31]

CLAIMS FOR (UNVERIFIED)

Alan W. Bell, Alfacell's public relations firm, issued a press release promoting Pannon as a cancer cure. It stated that clinical studies were on-going and would be verified by prestigious investigators at the site of the trials in the Dominican Republic.

CLAIMS AGAINST

On May 10, 1985, the U.S. Food and Drug Administration ordered Alfacell to cease exporting Pannon, claiming that Alfacell had shipped Pannon to the Dominican Republic illegally.

There are suspicions that Alfacell's frequent press releases are manipulating the stock market; rumors of takeovers and short selling by insiders can probably be credited for the stock's volatile performance. One anonymous Alfacell executive does say that the company is over-promoting itself. Stock once jumped from twelve dollars to twenty-three dollars after an announcement of clinical trials.[32]

Pharmacological Therapies

A number of different alternative drugs have been used in the treatment of rheumatoid arthritis. These drugs, used for the treatment of other ailments, have been found to be moderately effective in relieving the symptoms of arthritis.

These drugs include:

- dapsone
- pyrithioxine
- tiopronin
- thiopyridoxine
- haloperidol
- ethylenediaminetetraacetate (EDTA)
- captopril
- cisretinoic acid
- thalidomide
- isoprinoside

CLAIMS FOR

The use of dapsone has shown significant improvement in rheumatoid arthritis symptoms, both clinically and in the laboratory.

Pyrithioxine, tiopronin and thiopyridoxine have been studied in numerous trials as replacements for penicillamine. These drugs were tested to determine if their toxicity level was lower than the penicillamine. They showed average to significant improvement in symptoms.

Haloperidol, a tranquilizer, provided average improvement in patients. Ethylenediaminetetraacetate provided good improvement in symptoms. Captopril, cisretinoic acid, thalidomide, and isoprinoside all showed average improvement in arthritis symptoms.

CLAIMS AGAINST

None of the drugs have been tested extensively enough to

be regarded as antirheumatics. With all of the listed drugs, side effects were frequent. Further testing is required before they can be legitimately accepted for use.

Dapsone had potentially serious side effects, including anemia, headache, and possibly agranulocytosis. Ethylenediaminetetraacetate showed toxic reactions including nausea and potassium loss.

Tetracycline

Antimicrobial drugs have been used to treat patients with rheumatoid arthritis. This use was based on the theory that arthritis was caused by a bacterial, spirochete, or viral infection. In addition to tetracycline, rifamycin, ceftriaxone and ampicillin were all used for testing as well. Tetracycline was used for treatment based on the theory that arthritis was caused by mycoplasma infection.

CLAIMS FOR

If arthritis is caused by an infection, the symptoms and the ailment can be treated by using antimicrobial drugs. In a double-blind trial, patients with chronic inflammatory arthritis were given 2 gm/day of ceftriaxone intravenously for two weeks. Results were encouraging in about 40% of the patients.

Use of ampicillin at 3 gm/day for three months during the first year of disease followed by traditional drugs such as antimalarials or gold showed retardation of progression in 58% of the patients. Up to 16% showed complete remission after 4½ years.

Current trials are underway to determine if other antimicrobials, such as minocycline, are effective in treating rheumatoid arthritis.

CLAIMS AGAINST

There is no evidence that rheumatoid arthritis or any other inflammatory arthritis is caused by infectious agents. There have been no peer-reviewed journal articles that have shown that any antimicrobial agents have any effect on these diseases.

In several treatment centers, tetracycline derivatives have been advocated for treatment of rheumatoid arthritis. The early suggestions of benefit are thought not to be due to antibiotic effects but rather to inhibition of synovial collagenase. It is believed that such inhibition might limit tissue damage.

Clinical trials using aminoglycosidal antibiotics for arthritis showed minimal benefit while the side effects were numerous and serious.[33]

Chapter 4

DIETARY THERAPIES

71 / General Dietary Information
73 / Macrobiotic Diets
77 / Megadose Vitamin Theory

DIETARY THERAPIES

General Dietary Information

There is no universal diet that will work for every person. Because each body is different, a diet will affect each person differently. There have been a number of claims for different diets, whether to cure ailments or to assist in weight-loss.

The Saint Barnabas Medical Center in New Jersey studied dietary eliminations for their effect on arthritis. It eliminated such items as:

- red meat
- additives
- preservatives
- fruit
- dairy products
- herbs
- spices
- alcohol

When the tests were concluded, the center reported that there was no consistent effect on the disease. These tests, while they showed that diet had no significant effect on arthritis, did indicate that some sufferers may experience increased symptoms because of the foods that they eat.

There is a possibility that some foods react improperly with the body's immune system, causing the immune system to assume that they are invaders. This would cause an uncontrolled immune response.

Studies have also shown that there may be links between the development of arthritis and the consumption of wheat, corn, or beef products, but these links are isolated and have never been proven.

Fasting may provide temporary relief from arthritic pain, but has serious health consequences if followed for extended periods.

Tests of nutritional supplements have resulted in either negative or inconsistent results. Some supplements have caused irreversible disease and impairment as a result of extended use.

In the past few years, twenty-seven people died of eosinophilia myalgia syndrome from using amino acid products through a nutritional supplement. This is a white blood cell disease that impairs the nervous and muscular systems.

It is most important to consult with a physician before embarking on a dietary change. Patients should discuss their intentions and keep the physician informed of any additional changes they intend to make.

Drastic changes in diet often cause more problems than they solve.

Exhaustive testing and data collection have been performed to determine the effects of diet and dietary supplements on the incidence of cancers in both animals and humans. The information gathered from surveys and clinical studies has shown that the greatest preventive measure is a diet rich in vitamins obtained from fruit and vegetables.

While supplementary vitamins provided some additional protection, their effect was most noticeable in those people whose diets did not include a high intake of fruits and vegetables since the natural source of vitamins was not present.

Throughout numerous tests performed to determine the effects of vitamins on lung cancer patients, the incidence of lung cancer increased with the addition of beta-carotene, but decreased modestly with an increased intake of fruit and vegetables.

Current studies are attempting to determine the reasons for a marked difference in cancer occurrence or reduction due to diet. Something in the composition of raw fruits and vegetables allows the body to assimilate the vitamins quickly and easily, whereas supplements do not seem to provide the same function.

All studies of vitamin impact indicate inconclusive results and state the need for additional study to determine effects.

Macrobiotic Diets

In the 1960s, George Oshawa introduced macrobiotic diets to North America. He lectured across the United States on these diets, which originated in Japan, claiming that to treat and prevent cancers, diets are to be varied according to the Yin and Yang nature of the tumors.

This is a dietary system derived from Zen Buddhism and consisting chiefly of organically grown fruits, vegetables, and fish. It is usually accompanied by brown rice. This diet is believed to extend life.

Oshawa's proposal for health was the use of ten diets, each being more restrictive than the previous. One of the most restrictive diets, diet number seven, is recommended as the ideal for health. It consists entirely of cereals. For all these diets, liquids must be taken sparingly.

CLAIMS FOR

Anthony J. Sattilaro, M.D., an anesthesiologist at Methodist Hospital in Philadelphia has stated that this diet cured him of metastatic prostate cancer.

The macrobiotic diet and lifestyle have been recommended not only for cancer treatment, but also for cancer prevention.[1]

Kushi, a medical researcher, claims that cancer results from behavior, not only through improper diet, but also through mental attitude and lifestyle. Kushi believes that poor diet causes a toxic blood condition and that cancer is a natural mechanism for detoxifying the body. He therefore believes it imperative not to remove or destroy the cancer; he claims radiation therapy, chemotherapy, and surgery are toxic and violent therapies which hinder the recovery of macrobiotically treated patients.[2]

Once a practitioner has made a macrobiotic diagnosis, he puts the patient on a specific diet in the belief that the appropriate dietary treatment will restore balance and thus resolve the cancerous state.[3]

CLAIMS AGAINST

Literature searches by the American Cancer Society (ACS) Medical Library found no studies on macrobiotic diets as a method for either preventing or treating cancer.

Mr. Kushi provided no evidence to support his claims that patients who have undergone surgery, radiation, or chemotherapy will not respond well to a macrobiotic diet. He has discouraged the use of all conventional therapies, with the result that patients tend to avoid them. He has not responded to requests by the American Cancer Society for documentation of his claims.[4]

The safety and adequacy of the macrobiotic diet in cancer treatment cannot be accurately verified because of a lack of relevant scientific data. There are no descriptive studies of the clinical progress of cancer patients following the use of macrobiotic diets. There are also no records of controlled trials of the diet in animals. Many patients reporting "miraculous" cures had been receiving conventional medical therapy at the same time.

Two surveys of the dietary intakes of macrobiotic children and adults have been published. Some of the results were as follows:

- The diets were low in calories—most of the healthy adults reported having lost weight on the diet.
- Several cases of protein-calorie malnutrition have

been documented among infants and children who were fed strict macrobiotic diets.

- An adult woman who had followed diet number seven for eight months had lost thirty-five pounds and on hospitalization was near death with the classical manifestations of scurvy and severe folic acid and protein deficiency.
- Several cases of nutritional rickets have been documented in macrobiotic children.
- Intakes of riboflavin, niacin, vitamin B and folate were below the recommended dietary allowance (RDA).
- Calcium intakes in macrobiotic adults and children were 50-60% below the RDA.
- Iron intakes of macrobiotic women and children averaged 62-84% of the RDA; those of men exceeded the RDA.

The standard macrobiotic diet consists of 50-60% whole cereal grains. Allergic reactions caused by eating cereals may cause:

- gastrointestinal disturbances
- vomiting
- diarrhea
- bloating
- eczema
- urticaria
- angioedema
- asthma
- anaphylactic shock

Because of the high fibre content of the macrobiotic diet, there is a risk of complete obstruction in the presence of a narrowed intestinal lumen.

The Council of Foods and Nutrition of the American Medical Association and the Committee on Nutrition of the American Academy of Pediatrics, concerned that the more restrictive macrobiotic diets are nutritionally inadequate, have emphatically condemned them. The councils warn that effects of strict adherence to the diets could include scurvy, anemia, hypoproteinemia, hypocalcemia, emaciation due to starvation, loss of kidney function due to reduced fluid intake, other forms of malnutrition, and even death.[5]

Megadose Vitamin Therapy

Megadose vitamin therapy is also known as ortho-molecular therapy.

The popularity of vitamin megadoses reached a peak in the 1970s. These doses were usually twenty to six hundred times the recommended daily allowance, or 100 mg to 5 g/day. The practice became extensive because vitamins can be easily obtained over the counter.

Sales of vitamin supplements in health food stores in 1990 were estimated at $750 million. Sales at pharmacies were considerably higher.

CLAIMS FOR

There have been many studies performed to determine whether vitamins can play a role in cancer prevention. These epidemiologic studies have shown, for example, that vitamin C and vitamin E will provide significant protective effect.

Antioxidant micronutrients are one of the body's primary defenses against free radicals and reactive oxygen molecules. Vitamin C, vitamin E, and carotenoids trap these molecules and help prevent cancers. While these studies provide strong evidence of protection in animal studies, the effects on humans are less obvious. This is probably due to inconsistent or improper methods used in assessing the effects of diet on human cancers in epidemiological studies.

There are many indicators that vitamin C will provide protective effects for cancers of the esophagus, oral cavity, stomach, pancreas, cervix, rectum and breast. There was even substantial evidence that vitamin C would assist in the reduction of lung cancer.

Tests were performed on hamsters with kidney tumors induced by estradiol or diethylstilbestrol. It was determined that vitamin C reduced the incidence of induced cancer by almost 50%, but did not influence the growth of hormone dependent kidney tumors.

It is possible that vitamin C can inhibit tumorigenesis by decreasing concentrations of chemicals and DNA adducts that cause tumors.

Evidence of the protective effect of vitamins in preventing non-hormone dependent cancers is strong. It is noted that ascorbic acid, carotenoids, synthetic retinoids, beta-carotene, folic acid, choline/methionine, zinc, vitamin C, vitamin A and selenium have shown considerable effect. Increased consumption of fruits and vegetables are encouraged as a method of obtaining adequate supplies of these vitamins.

There is evidence that Filipino people who regularly chew the betel nut may benefit from the effects of dietary retinol (vitamin A) and/or carotene (provitamin A) derived from the nut. It is possible that these components may be factors in the prevention of oral cancer, which has a high rate of occurrence in Asia.[6]

It is possible that vitamins A, C, E, and folate may hinder the development of cancer. Vitamin A may cause precancerous cells to return to normal, while vitamins C and E may block the formation of carcinogens from food substances. It is important that any vitamin supplements be prescribed by a doctor since megadoses of some vitamins may be poisonous.[7]

One theory that may explain vitamin C's effectiveness against cancer and other cell-proliferative diseases states that ascorbic acid is required for the synthesis of a physiological inhibitor which normally prevents cells from depolymerizing the highly viscous intercellular glycosaminoglycans which restrain them.[8]

A study of fifty advanced cancer patients who were administered large doses of vitamin C showed that the vitamin enhanced natural resistance to cancer, even though the patients were terminal and "untreatable." The researchers expressed their expectation that patients in the earlier stages of cancer would benefit even more.[9]

Cameron (a medical researcher) reported a case in which a forty-two-year-old man with reticulum cell sarcoma treated only with large doses of ascorbic acid experienced complete regression.[10]

Researchers Cameron and Pauling, studying one hundred terminal cancer patients who had been treated with supplemental vitamin C versus one thousand matched controls, concluded that survival rates were greater for the patients who had received the supplement. On average, those patients lived three hundred days longer that did their controls. Twenty-two percent of them had survival times greater than one year after the date of untreatability as compared to 0.4% for the controls. Those twenty-two were still alive 2.4 years after reaching the apparently terminal stage, and eight were still alive after 3.5 years.[11]

CLAIMS AGAINST

While considerable animal studies have been done to determine the effects of vitamins in reducing the incidence of cancer, there are very few reliable test results from human cases. *In vitro* studies have shown some association between the use of vitamins C and E in the reduction of carcinogenic nitrosamines, but the evidence is not conclusive. More standardized and carefully controlled experiments are necessary to properly and adequately evaluate the use of vitamins in cancer treatment or prevention.

Although vitamins have been available for a long time, only recently have they been proclaimed for use as advanced cancer treatments. Self-prescribed megadoses as preventatives or as treatments for cancer can be potentially harmful.[12]

Widespread abuse of vitamin supplements has resulted because of claims by some scientists and physicians that vitamin megadoses can cure specific illnesses and because of commercial exploitation by pharmaceutical companies and health food fad stores.[13]

It is important to realize that while some vitamin therapies are being used as scientifically based cancer treatments, others are as yet unproven.[14]

Moertel conducted a double-blind study of one hundred and fifty people with advanced cancer to determine if there were any benefits in high-dose vitamin C treatments. None of the patients showed any effects to symptoms, performance, appetite or weight. All of the patients had a median survival of seven weeks. The researchers concluded that they were unable to prove any therapeutic benefits to the treatments.[15]

Pauling, one of the researchers who had determined that there was benefit to be gained from the use of vitamin C, criticized the results of the study, claiming that vitamin C was unable to stimulate the host defenses because all of the patients had received chemotherapy.[16]

Moertel decided to do a second double-blind study on one hundred patients who had not received chemotherapy. He selected patients with advanced colorectal cancer and, by random selection, assigned them either a vitamin C treatment or a placebo. Again, as in the first study, he found that none of the patients had any objective improvements. He determined that there was no difference between the groups in either the progression of the disease or on eventual survival intervals. On the basis of his findings, he concluded that high-dose vitamin C treatments were ineffective against cancer.[17]

Vitamin A

A proper diet contains about 5,000 to 10,000 International Units (IU) per day. Taking 25,000 to 50,000 IU per day for eight months or longer could be toxic. A single enormous dose of 1,500,000 IU is enough to poison an adult. This type of acute poisoning causes:

- drowsiness
- headache
- vomiting
- papilledema

Researchers have found that some patients with vitamin A intoxication showed psychiatric complications such as depression, irritability, and malaise; in one patient vitamin A was suspected of causing confusion, rapid weight gain and distorted thinking. These symptoms disappeared on discontinuing the megadoses of vitamin A. One patient had been taking 1,000,000 International Units of vitamin A for several weeks.[18]

A four-year-old boy with minimal brain dysfunction who was given massive doses of vitamin A by his grandmother suffered four months of fever and irritability and subsequently showed an abnormal bone scan and abnormal liver function.[19]

Vitamin B$_6$ (Pyridoxine)

Studies show that doses of several grams daily for prolonged periods can result in severe damage to nerves, loss of coordination, numbness around the mouth, and clumsiness of the hands and feet. Neurological studies of afflicted patients showed serious loss of limb reflexes and position and vibration sense as well as profound impairment of the ability to feel pain, temperature, and touch.[20]

Vitamin C

A study in which high doses of vitamin C were given to hamsters being exposed to various carcinogens showed the vitamin may inhibit tumor induction in the respiratory tract and in the nasal cavities, but that it seemed to accelerate the development of tumors in the larynx and trachea.[21]

While studying the effects of metal solutions on human cells, Dr. Robert Whiting of the B.C. Cancer Research Centre discovered that large doses of vitamin C could be carcinogenic.

Studies show that excessive ingestion of vitamin C can cause kidney stones and that dosages of 4 grams (4,000 mg) per day increased the level of a chemical called oxalate in the urine.

Dr. Hans Stich, head of the B.C. Cancer Research Centre Environmental Carcinogenic Unit reported that vitamin C can cause genetic damage to the cells, both of bacteria and mammals.

Commonly prescribed drugs can be affected by some vitamins. Vitamin C, for instance, may decrease the effect of oral anticoagulants, cause increased serum concentration, and, when taken with oral contraceptives, cause adverse effects of estrogen.[22]

Studies have shown that megadoses of vitamin C destroy significant amounts of vitamin B_{12} in the patient's regular diet and may lead to a deficiency of that vitamin.[23]

Vitamin D

Taking doses of 60,000 IU or more per day can cause:

- hypercalcemia (elevated calcium levels) with muscle weakness
- apathy
- headache

- anorexia
- nausea and vomiting
- bone pain
- ectopic calcification (calcium deposits other than in the bones)
- proteinuria (abnormal protein in urine)
- hypertension (elevated blood pressure)
- cardiac arrhythmia (irregular heart beat)

Vitamin E

Although people have taken relatively large doses of vitamin E for extended periods without apparent harm, researchers reported that 300 to 800 IU per day occasionally caused muscle weakness, fatigue, headaches, and nausea. One study showed intestinal cramps and diarrhea resulted from doses of 3200 IU per day for seven to nine weeks. Apparently, large doses of vitamin E can antagonize vitamin K and cause an increase in blood clotting time, as well as increase the effects of oral anticoagulants. One physician reported his practice had cured six cases of newly diagnosed hypertension by discontinuing large doses of vitamin E.[24]

Vitamin K

Taking large amounts of vitamin K while pregnant can cause jaundice in newborn children. High vitamin K supplements can block the effects of oral anticoagulants.

Niacin (Nicotinic acid)

Niacin causes release of histamine which in turn can

cause severe flushing, itching and gastrointestinal disturbances. In one trial, three grams of niacin daily increased serum uric acid and fasting blood glucose concentrations.

Large doses of niacin can cause liver toxicity. Increased aminotransferase activity (liver enzyme released when the liver is damaged) occurs frequently, and cholestatic jaundice (obstruction of the bile ducts in the liver) that disappears when the vitamin is discontinued has been reported with as little as 750 mg daily taken for less than three months.

Chapter 5

HERBAL THERAPIES

89 / Chapparal
90 / Comfrey
93 / Essential Oils
95 / Essiac
98 / Feverfew
99 / Ginseng
102 / Harry Hoxsey's Herbal Tonic
103 / Herbal Teas
108 / Iscador
110 / Sassafras
111 / Taheebo
113 / Valerian

HERBAL THERAPIES

Chapparal

Chaparral tea is an old Indian cure made by steeping the leaves and stems of the creosote bush. It has been researched at the University of Utah as an herbal for curing cancer.

CLAIMS FOR

A resident in surgery at the University of Utah, Dr. Hugh H. Hogle, presented a paper on chapparal tea for treating cancer at a meeting of the Utah Chapter of the American College of Surgeons. This presentation was published in the newspapers and resulted in international publicity and interest.

According to the University of Utah, some patients responded to treatment with chapparal tea. Two of these had melanoma (cancer arising from a mole), one had choriocarcinoma (cancer arising from pregnancy tissue) which had spread to the lungs, and one had lymphosarcoma (a malignant tumor of the lymphatic system).

Further, researchers cited the case of an eighty-five-year-old man with a malignant melanoma of the right cheek which had spread to his neck who refused surgery and treated himself with the tea and returned eight months later with marked regression of the cancer.[1]

CLAIMS AGAINST
The National Cancer Institute in the United States tested chapparal *in vitro* (in an artificial environment). These tests showed that it was very effective against cancer. However, when it was tested *in vivo* (in a living body) it failed the cancer chemotherapy tests. The American Cancer Society carefully studied all of the literature and information regarding chapparal and the tests performed with it, both *in vitro* and *in vivo*.

They determined that the tests do not show any evidence that the use of chapparal tea has any benefit in treating cancer in human beings.

Chapparal has an active ingredient called nordihydro-guaiaretic acid (NDGA). Tests have shown that this ingredient is very toxic, and long-term studies in rats caused lesions in the mesenteric lymph nodes and kidneys.

The U.S. Food and Drug Administration has removed chapparal from its "generally recognized as safe" (GRAS) list.

Comfrey

Comfrey (or Russian Comfrey) is the common name for the herb *Symphytum officinale*. The active ingredient is allantoin which is found in the roots and leaves. Comfrey may also be known as blackwort or knitbone.

CLAIMS FOR (UNVERIFIED)

Historically, comfrey was used in the sixteenth century for healing wounds, inflammation, gout, ulcers, and gangrene. According to proponents, it is used in the modern world for healing malignancies (cancers). It is claimed to be useful for treating:

- pulmonary hemorrhages
- diarrhea
- dysentery
- internal ulcers
- glandular disorders
- chronic cough
- bronchitis
- gout
- hoarseness
- sore gums
- varicose veins
- inflammations
- burns
- sores
- sprains
- fractures
- gangrene
- otitis
- mastitis
- fibrositis
- pleurisy

CLAIMS AGAINST

Pyrrolizidine alkaloids, the major active ingredients in comfrey, can be found in many different types of plants. The Senecio species of alkaloid has been found in *Symphytum officinale*. Studies have revealed that the pyrrolizidine alkaloids—senkirkine and symphatine—caused liver tumors in rats.

Controlled studies on rats injected with *Symphytum officinale* have shown that the plant is carcinogenic. Earlier studies had already demonstrated the carcinogenicity of ingested comfrey roots and leaves.[2]

Since the pyrrolizidine alkaloids which are present in all forms of *Symphytum officinale* are toxic and have been known to cause tumors, neither humans nor animals should consume comfrey in any form.

Data on the effects of pyrrolizidine alkaloids in animals is readily available, but reliable human data is scarce because the effects of chronic poisoning do not appear for several years. Because of this delay, the cause cannot be easily isolated or recognized. The most reliable report involves a group of approximately seven thousand people who had eaten food made with contaminated flour. Their estimated consumption was 2 mg/day of pyrrolizidine alkaloids. Within two years, 23% of the people had severe liver impairment.

The continuous consumption of comfrey root tea will cause serious health problems. One cup of comfrey tea can have 8-26 mg of pyrrolizidine alkaloids.

Food supplements containing *Symphytum* from comfrey can be found in many health-food stores. These are usually in the form of comfrey-pepsin capsules or tablets sold as digestive aids. Users are instructed to take them daily over long periods of time or even permanently.

In one case, a forty-nine-year-old woman who had been taking the capsules regularly was diagnosed with Veno-occlusive disease in a form of Budd-Chiari syndrome (obstruction of the veins in the liver). Chemical analysis of the contents of the capsules revealed the presence of pyrrolizidine alkaloids. Doctors estimated she had consumed approximately 85 mg of the alkaloids. Her tests results indicated chronic pyrrolizidine intoxication, leading researchers to suspect that low-level chronic exposure to the alkaloids had caused her veno-occlusive disease.[3]

Essential Oils

Essential oils are derived from plant leaves, stems, or roots. These oils are usually distilled or cold-extracted and their active ingredients are extremely concentrated. They are prized for their potency and are used as remedies for a number of ailments. The most common oils are evening primrose oil and oil of anise.

Evening primrose is a stout, erect American biennial herb of the genus *Oenothera biennis*. It has conspicuous yellow flowers which open in the evening. The active ingredient is linoleic acid, a colourless to yellow oily fatty acid. This acid ($C_{18}H_{32}O_2$) is also found in linseed oil, cottonseed oil, and other vegetable oils.

Capsules of evening primrose oil have been found to have a high concentration of borage oil. Borage is an erect rough European herb of the genus *Borago officinalis*. It has blue flowers and includes such plants as forget-me-not, alkanet, and heliotrope. Alkanet is used to make red dye.

Anise is a small South European and North African plant of the genus *Pimpinella anisum*. The fragrant seed of the plant is used in cooking and for flavorings.

CLAIMS FOR (UNVERIFIED)

Evening primrose oil contains high concentrations of linoleic acid, gamma-linoleic acid and vitamin E. Gamma-linoleic acid (GLA) is an essential fatty acid that the body requires but does not manufacture. It can only be obtained through food.

Evening primrose oil (GLA) alleviates the pain and inflammation caused by arthritis. It also prevents the following:

- hardening of the arteries
- heart disease
- premenstrual syndrome
- multiple sclerosis
- high blood pressure

In addition, GLA has a positive effect on hormone response, lowers cholesterol levels, aids in treating cirrhosis of the liver and relieves pain and inflammation.

Oil of anise relieves pain and inflammation caused by arthritis.

CLAIMS AGAINST

The presence of linoleic acid does not indicate that GLA necessarily is also present. The linoleic acid must convert to GLA to be of any value. A random sampling of capsules containing evening primrose oil was tested for content. Of sixteen capsules tested, fourteen contained gamma-linoleic acid. Concentration levels varied from

7% to 10%. The remainder of the contents were determined to be borage oil.

In a six-month double-blind test, forty patients with rheumatoid arthritis were tested using evening primrose oil. The placebo was olive oil. All patients continued to receive non-steroidal anti-inflammatory medication. Of the forty patients, twenty-one received primrose oil and nineteen received olive oil. In each group, three patients reduced their dosage of anti-inflammatory drugs. Patients on evening primrose oil showed a reduction in morning stiffness at three months, but patients on olive oil showed a reduction in pain and articular index after six months. The results of the test indicate that the evening primrose oil did not exceed the results of olive oil.

In a double-blind placebo-controlled trial with patients suffering from primary liver cancer, no statistically significant effects were observed on survival time or liver size.

Ingestion of oil of anise in small quantities can cause nausea, vomiting, convulsions, and fluid in the lungs.

Essiac

Essiac is an herbal remedy given to Nurse Rene Caisse by native North American Indians. Nurse Caisse, from Bracebridge, was convinced that the remedy would be effective against cancer. The name of the preparation is taken from "Caisse" spelled backwards. Her story was published in Toronto's *Homemaker's Magazine*. It resulted in a great deal of public interest and in scientific investigation.

Essiac is a tea made from four dried herbs—Indian rhubarb, sheephead sorrel, slippery elm, and burdock. It is manufactured by the Resperin Corporation in Toronto, Canada.

CLAIMS FOR (UNVERIFIED)

Throughout the 1920s and 1930s, Rene Caisse defied the medical establishment and treated hundreds of cancer patients (most of them terminal) with her secret herbal cure. She apparently produced remarkable results.

CLAIMS AGAINST

In a later issue following the original Caisse story, *Homemaker's Magazine* noted that the two doctors who originally tested Essiac had stated that they could find no evidence to support the belief that it would cure cancer. They had studied sixty cases where the preparation had been given to cancer patients and could determine no alteration in the progression of the disease.

Dr. K. J. R. Wightman, medical director of the Ontario Cancer Treatment and Research Foundation and a former president of the Royal College of Physicians and Surgeons commented that while he acknowledged the furore that Essiac had caused, Nurse Caisse's preparation had no effect at all on the disease process of any patients tested with the substance. Some subjective improvements were noted, but they could well have been the result of a placebo effect. Wightman reported that in one trial, eighteen out of forty patients had died and a further fifteen were withdrawn because of definite deterioration. Four patients with very slowly progressing disease had shown no response. The remaining three patients with chronic lymphatic leukemia (cancer of the blood-producing bone marrow) had also experienced no change in any parameter of their disease status. Another study of twenty-five more patients showed similar results. Wightman concluded that the evidence was overwhelmingly against any claims of Essiac's effectiveness.[4]

The Health Protection Branch (Canada) contacted 150 physicians who were known to have received supplies of Essiac from Resperin Corporation in Toronto. Replies from seventy-four of the physicians revealed that of eighty-six patients, forty-seven reported no benefits, seventeen had died, one had subjective improvement, five required less pain relief, four had objective response, four were in stable condition, and eight reports were not evaluable. Of the eight who either had objective response or were in stable condition, three were found upon reexamination by their physicians to have progression of the disease. The Health Protection Branch, upon reviewing further documentation of three who were in stable condition, decided that the stability was due to other forms of treatment. The Health Protection Branch then concluded that there was no proof that Essiac had helped in any way. However, the HPB approved the distribution of Essiac to physicians who felt there was no other effective treatment available and who felt their patients may benefit from a possible placebo effect.[5]

Rene Caisse refused to share her secret herbal remedy. Instead, she signed over the rights to the secret formula to the Resperin Corporation. There were many offers to help her achieve recognition and to provide for the distribution of Essiac, both from scientific groups and from laymen.

In 1936 the Banting Institute offered to provide Mrs. Caisse with mice inoculated with mouse sarcoma (malignancy arising from fibrous or connective tissue cells) and with chickens inoculated with Rouse sarcoma. The animals would be placed at her disposal in a laboratory so that she could perform the necessary tests. She did not even have to tell anyone the secret ingredients of the herbal remedy. She rejected the offer.

During the 1950s, Dr. Shields Warren of the U.S. National Cancer Institute suggested that they could do animal tests using the remedy. When Mrs. Caisse discovered that they would require the formula for the remedy, she rejected the offer.

In Sault Ste. Marie, Dr. D. Walde tested Essiac on forty patients with proven cancer. None of the patients showed any measurable improvement.

Essiac is currently a commercial venture that could stand to make considerable financial profit from marketing this herbal remedy if it can prove the remedy is effective in the treatment of cancer. By December 1985, the Resperin Corporation was charging ten dollars for a bottle of Essiac. The normal dosage is about three bottles per month for one to two years, sometimes longer. Patients must also pay for delivery by air courier service.

Feverfew

Feverfew is an erect bushy herb (*Chrysanthemum parthenium*) of the family Compositae. The plants of the Compositae family are the largest, most highly developed, and widely distributed in the vegetable kingdom. They are mostly herbaceous shrubs and trees. The flowers usually occur in dense clusters opening from a central cup-shaped envelope. Other plants in the family include dandelion, chrysanthemum, dahlia, and aster.

The active ingredients include alpha-methylbutyrolactones (lactone), borneol, camphor, parthenolide, pyrethrin, santamarine and terpene.

CLAIMS FOR (UNVERIFIED)

In addition to eliminating worms, stimulating appetite, increasing the fluidity of lung and bronchial tube mucus, and stimulating uterine contractions, feverfew will relieve the following:

- headache
- arthritis
- indigestion
- colds
- fever
- muscle tension

CLAIMS AGAINST

The effects of lactone and parthenolide are potentially toxic. These chemicals cause irreversible inhibition of the contractile responses of the aortic ring. Inhibition of the secretory activity of blood platelets also occurs.

Ginseng

True ginseng comes from the root of a perennial herb *Panax ginseng*, normally found in Eastern Asia. *Panax quinquefolium* can be found in Eastern U.S. and Canada, while *Panax pseudoginseng* is usually found in India, China and Japan.

While ginseng is normally associated with *Panax ginseng*, it can be used to refer to many different varieties of related plants. The principal active ingredient of ginseng is believed to be titerpenoid saponin. This compound is extremely confusing and complex and may even have different names. There are differences between oriental and American ginseng.

CLAIMS FOR

Ginseng has been used for thousands of years as a tonic and as a remedy for all types of illness. It has been described in detail by oriental folk medicine. It is still widely used in Chinese medicine as a stimulant to increase metabolism and to regulate blood pressure and blood glucose. The only recognized medical use in the United States is in skin ointments.

Ginseng has been hailed as a healthful tonic, stimulant, and aphrodisiac (substance which will increase sexual performance). There may be over five million ginseng users in the United States. Other claims maintain that ginseng will increase resistance to cancer and assist cancer patients to recover.

One study on ginseng as a cancer cure reported that a twenty-six-year-old patient with chronic myelocytic (arising from the granulated white blood cells) leukemia had her clinical symptoms disappear. Her laboratory findings returned to normal except for her leucocyte number and LDH value (LDH is an enzyme released when liver cells are damaged). Researchers concluded that the remission was due to the enhancement of the host-resistance.[6]

Researchers tested ginseng to evaluate its ability to prevent and to cure cancer. In one such test, using red ginseng on newborn mice, they found that ginseng extract seems to inhibit the growth of lung cancers caused by environmental carcinogens such as urethane, dimethyl benzanthracene, and aflatoxin B_1. They concluded that further research may prove the extract could be used as a preventative or delaying agent for these kinds of cancers.[7]

When testing whether ginseng would prevent infections in mice, researchers found that treated mice responded by forming antibodies in direct relation to dosage. The most pronounced effect was that killer-cell activity was increased by as much as 44% to 150% depending on the effect-to-target cell ratios used in the assay. Test showed that *in vitro*, ginseng inhibited lymphocyte proliferation and enhanced interferon production. *In vivo*, however, although tests showed enhanced interferon production, they could not show comparable inhibition of lymphocyte proliferation.[8]

CLAIMS AGAINST

Ginseng has estrogens (female hormones). They can cause swollen and painful breasts. Other substances such as mandrake root are often sold as ginseng. Mandrake root contains scopolamine and reserpine.

Siegel observed that ginseng users suffer from intoxications (chronic insomnia, nervousness, and loose stools) requiring clinical attention.

There are more than twenty plants which are often referred to as ginseng. While some of these are members of the same plant family, others are completely unrelated. Because of these variations there is no standard combination of active ingredients.

No tests have been performed to determine if there is a potential abuse syndrome related to these plants. There have also been no clinical tests done to determine what the effects of ginseng are on the human body. These plants should not be used indiscriminately.

Obtaining authentic ginseng is rarely possible, as has been verified by independent studies. One analysis of 534 ginseng products showed that 60% of them were completely worthless and that 25% of them contained absolutely no ginseng. It is interesting to note that the genuine product is extremely expensive, often selling for more than $20 per ounce. The high cost of true "Korean Red" ginseng and the complete lack of quality control over distributors have resulted in a variety of products (including teas, powders, tablets, extracts, and other forms) which have an amazing variety of ingredients, the least of which is actually ginseng.[9]

Harry Hoxsey's Herbal Tonic

Harry Hoxsey's cancer treatment was based on a formula of ten weeds growing in a field. Apparently his grandfather's horse had grazed in the field and been cured of a reported leg cancer. After being prosecuted for violating the medical practice laws in several states, Hoxsey set up a clinic in Dallas, Texas. His treatment is still in use at the Biomedical Center in Tijuana.

CLAIMS FOR (UNVERIFIED)
Harry Hoxsey maintained that he cured external cancer

with a paste and internal cancers with an herbal drink. This concoction consisted of a combination of prickly ash, buckthorn, cascara, potassium iodide, alfalfa, red clover, and sugar syrup.

CLAIMS AGAINST

The U.S. Food and Drug Administration investigated at least four hundred cases of persons whom Hoxsey claimed to have cured of cancer by using his treatment. No case of a real cure was ever found. His clinic was closed in 1960 after legal battles which lasted ten years.

It is estimated that cancer patients paid over fifty million dollars to Harry Hoxsey for his tonic. Most of those patients died of their disease.

Herbal Teas

There are many different combinations of herbs used to make teas. Claims have been made that herbal teas may be used for both prevention and treatments.

CLAIMS FOR (UNVERIFIED)

There are many records from the ancient civilizations of Sumer, Assyria, Egypt, Greece, China, and Rome indicating that there are numerous special plants believed to possess medicinal qualities. These records show that thousands of plants have been considered medicines with the power to cure or prevent many different illnesses and afflictions.

CLAIMS AGAINST

None of the herbal teas have been shown to cure cancer;

many contain toxic and even cancer-causing substances. Most plant products sold by health food stores and by natural product distributors to be used for beverage purposes were never meant to be ingested. Almost all of those plants have been dropped from official practice in North America as either ineffective or harmful.

Many individual plants have physiologically active or toxic factors. They are often packaged singly or in combinations with other plants and carry no warning of chemical properties or possible side effects. Because every plant is different and the chemistry of each plant is variable, there is no such thing as a measured dose.

Specific geographical areas seem to have unusually high incidences of esophageal cancer. Researchers have spent considerable time trying to determine the causes and have found definite correlations between esophageal cancer and the use of native plant products. The drinking of herbal teas, especially, seems to be linked to the incidence of cancer. The following reports illustrate some other effects of drinking herbal teas:

CASE #1

A twenty-five-year-old woman with menometrorrhagia (abnormal uterine bleeding with heavy periods and bleeding between periods), was found to have an abnormally high blood clotting time. For years this woman had eaten only natural foods, and she had been drinking large quantities of an herbal tea. Three of the ingredients in her tonic were tonka beans, melilot, and sweet woodruff—all of them natural coumarins, or blood thinners.[10]

CASE #2

An Indian man who had experienced remission of his psoriasis while drinking an herbal tea passed the tea on to four young Chinese women who also suffered from the skin condition. One of these women subsequently developed a skin rash and discontinued drinking the tea. The other three women were admitted to hospital because they developed abdominal ascites (abnormal fluid in the abdominal cavity) and hepatomegaly (enlarged liver). Liver biopsies of all four women showed hepatic veno-occlusive disease. Other tests revealed ascites, oozing, enlarged esophageal veins and bloody mucous in the stomach. One of the women, the only one who continued drinking the tea, died eight weeks later from liver failure, high blood pressure, and gastrointestinal hemorrhage. When analyzed, the tea was found to contain chopped leaves, acorns, dates, seeds, sticks and cones. The leaves, which were of the family Compositae, contained pyrrolizidine alkaloids.[11]

CASE #3

A patient undergoing whole abdomen irradiation for ovarian cancer died of veno-occlusive disease of the liver. She had also been treated with herbal tea and chemotherapy, each of which may cause veno-occlusive disease. Physicians suspected her death was due to the interaction of these agents, something doctors should consider before prescribing combination treatments.[12]

CASE #4

Nerium oleander tea caused a young Los Angeles woman's death. She was admitted to hospital after complaining of vomiting and a numb tongue. Her pulse was weak and she appeared confused; her blood pressure was not palpable and she had an irregular heart beat. Her autopsy revealed pulmonary congestion and swelling and a mild thickening of the arteries. Her cause of death was listed as oleander intoxication.[13]

All parts of the oleander plant contain chemicals called cardiac glycosides (drugs similar to digitalis which is used as a powerful heart stimulant). These include oleandrin, oleandroside, nerioside and digitoxin. There is no way to deactivate these toxic compounds. Boiling or drying the plant does not affect their toxicity.

These chemicals will irritate mucous membranes in the mouth and cause bitter taste, nausea, vomiting, increased salivation, abdominal pain, and diarrhea. Central nervous system reactions will cause an altered mental status. Visual disturbances, such as dilation of the pupil, will occur. The chemicals will also cause painful nerves and weakness.

Juniper berries can irritate the gastrointestinal tract.

Shave grass or horsetail contains nicotine and thaminase. In horses and other grazing animals, these plants have caused excitement, loss of appetite and muscular control, diarrhea, labored breathing, convulsions, coma, and death.

Ingestion of half a cup of burdock root tea purchased in a health food store has resulted in blurred vision with enlarged pupils, dry mouth, inability to urinate, and bizarre behavior and speech, including hallucinations.

Nutmeg can cause hallucinations and very high doses can cause liver damage and death.

Camomile (Chamomile) tea may cause skin reactions, anaphylactic shock (severe wheezing and blood pressure drop—often fatal), and other severe hypersensitivity reactions in people allergic to ragweed, asters, chrysanthemums, or other members of the Compositae family.

The prolonged use of camomile tea and peppermint tea can result in clinical water intoxication and subsequent seizures because of inadequate sodium content.

Licorice root in large amounts can cause sodium and water retention, low blood potassium, high blood pressure, heart failure and cardiac arrest.

Devil's claw root can make the uterus contract and should be avoided during pregnancy.

Pennyroyal oil has caused death due to kidney and liver poisoning.

Indian tobacco, ingested in large quantities, can cause sweating, vomiting, paralysis, depressed temperature, coma and death.

The entire poke plant (pokeweed, inkberry) is toxic. Eating the uncooked plant can cause gastroenteritis, increased rate of breathing and death. Children have died from eating the berries.

Seeds, pits, bark or leaves of apricots, bitter almonds, some beans, cherries, choke cherries, peaches, pears, apples and plums contain compounds which liberate hydrogen cyanide. Adults have been poisoned by drinking milkshakes containing apricot kernels, and children have been poisoned and some have died after eating such seeds.

Goiter (enlarged thyroid gland), staggering gait, nerve damage, and blindness have all been linked to chronic cyanide poisoning caused by eating cassava.

Excessive consumption of aloe vera (which contains aloin) will cause severe diarrhea and cramps.

Chuifong Toukuwan, a Chinese herbal remedy for arthritis contains cortisone. This chemical will cause serious side effects.

The ingredients of some teas may be labelled incorrectly, and errors can occur in the correct identification of herbs by suppliers. This can create extremely hazardous health situations which could result in death.

Iscador

Iscador is made from various kinds of mistletoe, particularly those found growing on apple, fir, pine, oak, and elm trees. Its proper name is *Viscum album*.

Iscador was first proposed for the treatment of cancer in 1920 by Rudolf Steiner, founder of the Society for Cancer Research in Arlesheim, Switzerland. It was introduced into the treatment of human cancer as early as 1921. It was approved for use in Austria, Switzerland, and West Germany. It is also apparently being used in France, Holland, Eastern Europe, Britain, and Scandinavia.

CLAIMS FOR (UNVERIFIED)
The principal advocates of Iscador are:

Rita Leroi, M.D., President
Society for Cancer Research,
Arlesheim, Switzerland

Marvin I. Weinberger,
Belmont, Massachusetts

Henning Schramm, M.D.,

Weleda, Switzerland

According to the advocates, Iscador is recommended for treatment of inoperable tumors and for the preoperative treatment of tumors, for the therapy of solid tumors, and for precancerous conditions when indicated.

The rationale of Iscador treatment and the research on which it depends are based on the school of thought called "anthroposophy."

This concept of cancer states that an active principle called a "form-giving principle" lies behind cancer-controlling mechanisms.

Iscador is claimed to have special characteristics that inhibit tumor cell growth and enhance the controlling effect of the "form-giving organization" so that the tumor can be controlled.

Almost two million ampules of Iscador are sold annually in countries where it is prescribed. It is estimated that about thirty thousand patients are treated every year.

CLAIMS AGAINST

The Society for Cancer Research presented approximately seventeen clinical and chemical papers to the American Cancer Society about the effects of mistletoe extract on humans. The American Cancer Society submitted these papers to two expert consultants for evaluation. These consultants worked independently from each other, and their conclusions were that the documents presented no evidence that Iscador will prevent or cure human cancer.

The Society received from Mr. Weinberger a document titled "Iscador - a summary review." This document included clinical data and an extensive bibliography of twenty-five publications and fourteen unpublished manuscripts. This document was sent to the consultants to be evaluated. They indicated that there was little change from the material previously reviewed.

After careful study of the literature and other information available to it, the American Cancer Society does not have any evidence to substantiate the claim that cancer in human beings can be treated or prevented by Iscador. Lacking such evidence, the American Cancer Society strongly urges individuals afflicted with cancer not to participate in treatment with Iscador.

Iscador does not have the approval of the Food and Drug Administration. The active ingredient has not been identified, so the effects of the drug cannot be determined. There is no evidence that the treatments are effective.

Sassafras

This is the young root of sassafras or *Sassafras abdidum.* The active ingredient is safrole. Safrole is also a component of many essential oils, such as star anise oil, micranthum oil, and camphor oil.

Sassafras has been used for medicinal purposes as well as for beverages. The aromatic oil derived from the sassafras root bark has been used as a flavoring in soft drinks and in some pharmaceutical products.

The U.S. Food and Drug Administration banned sassafras after safrole was found to cause liver cancer.

CLAIMS AGAINST

Safrole is considered toxic in concentrations as low as 1%. It causes weight loss, shrinking of the testicles and bone marrow depletion. It also causes liver tumors.

Preliminary pharmacological experiments indicate that some liquid and alcoholic extracts of sassafras root bark can cause ataxia (loss of balance), ptosis (droopy eyelids), hypersensitivity to touch, central nervous system depression, and hypothermia (low body temperature). Safrole affects liver functions and will cause death if mixed with other drugs which can be broken down by the safrole.

Scientists studied effects of safrole on unborn and newborn mice by injecting the substance into the stomachs of pregnant and lactating mice. These young mice developed liver and kidney tumors in numbers high enough to suggest to researchers that safrole comes into contact with the fetus by crossing the placenta (organ that nourishes the fetus) and with infants through the mothers milk.[14]

Taheebo

Taheebo is the Indian name for the inner bark of the tabebuia tree, a genus of about one hundred broad-leaved, mostly evergreen trees found in the mountains of the Andes, the West Indies, Central and South America.

The active ingredient is lapachol, a yellow crystalline material also known as lapachic acid, taiguic acid, tecomin or green hartin.

A tea is prepared from the leaves or bark and is called taheebo tea, ipe roxo, red lapacho, lapacho avellendae, pau d'arco or tabebuia altissima.

CLAIMS FOR (UNVERIFIED)

Taheebo was used by the Inca Indians of South America one thousand years ago and is still used by the Callaway tribe, descendants of the Inca medicine men, to cure cancer and many other diseases.

Medical doctors in Argentina claim that taheebo will cure leukemia. Taheebo can also treat

- anemia (low red blood cells),
- arteriosclerosis (hardening and obstruction of the arteries),
- asthma,
- bronchitis,
- colitis (inflammation of the large bowel),
- diabetes,
- skin sores,
- gastritis (inflammation of the stomach), and
- infections.

CLAIMS AGAINST

In one series of recognized clinical trials, twenty-one patients were treated with lapachol. These included nineteen patients with advanced non-leukemic tumors and two patients with chronic myelocytic leukemia in relapse.

The doses of lapachol ranged from 250 to 3750 mg/day for five days. The largest total single dose was 3000 mg/day for twenty-one days. All of the patients had previously received a variety of different therapies which had failed to affect the cancer.

Only one woman benefitted from the lapachol; she had one osteoblastic (bone destroying) hip lesion improve, but all her other lesions remained unchanged. The other patients experienced either no change in their condition or became worse. Researchers discontinued the study because the very high doses of lapachol necessary caused nausea, vomiting and anticoagulation.[15]

The Canadian Federal Health Protection Branch banned taheebo in February 1985. This ban will remain in effect until distributors can prove it to be safe and effective. The plant also cannot be advertised or sold as a treatment, prevention, or cure for disease, including cancer.

Lapachol can inhibit the respiratory processes. Animal studies in which lapachol was administered orally showed that monkeys died after six doses of 0.5 g/kg/day and after five doses of 1.0 g/kg/day. Side effects in dogs and monkeys included anemia, reticulocytosis, normoblastosis, pallor of mucous membranes, bilirubinuria, and proteinuria. Dogs experienced transient thrombocytosis, leukocytosis, elevated serum alkaline phosphatase activity and blood clotting time.[16]

Valerian Root

Valerian is an old world perennial herb of the genus *Valeriana officinalis*. It has small pink or white flowers and a strong odour. In Japan, the root is called *Hokkai-Kisso*. It has traditionally been used as a carminative and sedative. Ingredients include acetic acid, butyric acid, emphene, chatinine, formic acid, glycosides, magnesium, volatile oils, valeric acid, and verine.

CLAIMS FOR (UNVERIFIED)

Valerian is good for nervousness, ulcers, headaches, colic, gas, pain, stress, anxiety, insomnia, convulsions, muscle cramps, and spasms. It improves circulation, aids in the relief of arthritis pain and reduces mucous from colds.

CLAIMS AGAINST

Valerian is a powerful sedative. In laboratory comparisons with diazepam and imipramine, the effects of valerian in decreasing spontaneous ambulation and inhibiting mobility were significantly higher. The results of laboratory testing indicate that valerian extract acts directly on the central nervous system. It is an antidepressant.

Laboratory testing shows minimal anticonvulsive properties.

Chapter 6

MISCELLANEOUS THERAPIES

117 / Definitions
119 / Alexander Technique
120 / Ayurvedic Medicine
122 / Crystals
124 / Homeopathic Therapies
128 / Network Chiropractic
129 / Reflexology

MISCELLANEOUS THERAPIES

Definitions

Therapies for disease and illness originate from many sources. Modern medicine has roots in ancient discovery as do alternative medicines. The difference is that modern medicine has advanced while alternative medicines have retained ancient beliefs and practices. Present-day life expectancy and control of disease would lead one to believe that modern medicine is more efficient and effective.

To better understand the therapies that fall into this category, you should know the definition of a few terms applied to alternative medicines.

HOLISM

Titus Lucretius Carus (100 – 55 B.C.) wrote in his collections of informative poetry that the body, mind and spirit were composed of many minute particles which were all formed together to create the body. This concept of small particles and subsystems synthesized together is considered holism, from which comes the adjective "holistic."

This belief states that you cannot affect one part of the body without affecting all parts, since there is no division. From holism come the concept of healing the body through meditation, attitude, faith, touching and the utilization of physical remedies.

HOMEOPATHY

This method of therapy is based on the belief that illness can be cured by using a remedy that under normal circumstances would cause the symptoms that you have from the illness. While this may seem confusing, it is best described as "like cures like." The difference is that the remedy is supplied in minute quantities. The belief is that the smaller the dose of the remedy, the more potent it is.

For example, mercury (in chemical form) is directly related to chronic inflammation and nervous system degradation, sore throats, and miscarriage. If you had any of the above symptoms, homeopathic medicine would prescribe a mercury cure.

NATUROPATHY

Naturopathic medicine advocates the use of the natural elements in healing. This is a drug-free method which uses only air, water, and sunshine for their natural effects. It also includes a regular program of exercise.

RELIGIOUS AND MYSTICAL THERAPIES

Religious medicines have formed the basis for healing since the dawn of time. These vary from the belief in the mystical healing powers of supreme beings to the powers of the elements of the earth.

Superstition as well as religion has also played a major part in alternative therapy. This can range from the addition of a ceramic rooster in the kitchen for good luck to the resonant alignment of your body elements in relation to crystals.

For example, there are beliefs that the remains of dead animals, once properly released from their earthly bonds, hold mystical healing powers. This involves a ceremony held under a full moon and the creation of "healing sticks" from the bones, skin, and feathers. Placed in your home or kept in the bed, these devices drive away disease and keep you safe from harm.

It is important to realize that many religious cures currently in vogue originated in China or India many centuries ago and have not changed since that time. That does not necessarily mean that they are effective or safe. On the other hand, there are many safe and effective natural remedies prescribed by these religious followings.

Alexander Technique

The Alexander technique was developed by an Australian actor, F. Matthias Alexander (1869-1955). He determined that his use of his body, in particular his stance, was causing chronic hoarseness when he performed.

Over a period of many years, Alexander developed his technique for correcting the misuse of the body. Alexander moved to London where he further developed his technique working with people who had specific physical problems, much to the amusement of the medical community.

The technique requires a qualified teacher to instruct the student in movement and stance so that he will have a more balanced body with increased efficiency. It is said to be a combination of yoga, massage, aerobics, physical therapy, self-hypnosis, biofeedback, transcendental meditation, and relaxation technique.

In 1994, group lessons cost about $60 U.S. for a six-week session while private lessons cost from $800 to $1200 U.S.

CLAIMS FOR (UNVERIFIED)
The therapy will cure neck and back pain, breathing problems and digestive disorders as well as muscular problems.

CLAIMS AGAINST
None.

Ayurvedic Medicine

Originating from ancient India, this medical treatise is a part of the Hindu religion. This religion worships Brahma as the supreme god who has a selection of lower gods ranked according to importance. The writings relating to the religion fall into four "vedas," with the medical writings considered to be the fifth veda. These writings form the basis of the Hindu scriptures and date back to 2000 B.C. Roughly translated, "veda" means "to know" and "ayur" means "span of life."

The vedas are:

Rigveda	sacrificial hymns
Yajurveda	doctrines and forms of worship
Samaveda	hymns to Indra, god of first rank
Aharvaveda	chants and incantations
Ayurveda	medical practice

The basic concept is that illness is caused by "doshas" or evil humors which govern the physiological and physicochemical activities of the body.

CLAIMS FOR (UNVERIFIED)

The chemicals and natural herbal remedies used in Ayurvedic medicine will assist in curing most illness, from cancer to epilepsy. Ginger is prescribed in Ayurvedic medicine as a cure for arthritis, rheumatism, and inflammation.

A study of fifty-six patients (twenty-eight with rheumatoid arthritis, eighteen with osteoarthritis and ten with muscular discomfort) who used powdered ginger, found that more than three-quarters of the arthritis patients found relief from pain and swelling, and that all the patients with muscular discomfort found relief from pain. None of them had harmful effects during the time of ginger consumption which lasted from three months to two and a half years.[1]

Ayurvedic practitioners use a process called "samskaras" to purify and detoxify natural remedies such as aconite, an extremely lethal substance from the genus *Aconitum*. This is a medicinal plant, commonly known as monkshood or wolfsbane. The poisonous active ingredient is acotine ($C_{34}H_{47}O_{11}N$) an alkaloid which forms flat white crystals.

Crude aconite is always purified through "samskaras" before being used in Ayurvedic medicines. A study done on mice to determine whether processed aconite is less toxic than the crude found 100% mortality in mice at a dose of 2.6 mg/mouse of crude aconite while there was no mortality at doses even eight times as high with the processed. The test also showed that all the steps in the processing were essential for complete detoxification.[2]

Ayurvedic medicine recommends regular application of sesame oil to the skin for prevention of skin disease. Tests have shown that sesame and safflower oils (containing linoleate) will inhibit the growth of malignant melanomas while coconut, olive and mineral oils (containing palmitic and oleic) will not.

CLAIMS AGAINST
The hazards of using herbal remedies remain constant. There is no way of knowing what the active ingredients are or what the concentration of those ingredients is. In addition, imported remedies often have other dangers.

Remedies from India have been found to contain heavy metals in high concentrations. One Indian patient with hepatitis actually contracted lead poisoning from an herbal remedy he was taking for diabetes.[3]

Crystals

Crystals have played an important part in ancient medicines. Tribal cultures used quartz crystals for their sacred powers. Chinese and Japanese Taoists believed that crystals had magic power and used them for contemplation and healing.

Modern-day believers, speaking from information which has been "channelled," or intuitively received, claim crystals provided energy for Atlantis. According to Judith Larkin, writing in *The Newcastle Guide to Healing With Crystals*, enormous crystals suspended under pyramids radiated energy to disc-shaped saucers for redirection.

Crystals were also used for thought projection and dematerialization and reconstruction of the body. This instantaneous method of travel was the standard in Atlantis. Quartz crystals implanted in the bases of the skulls of servants programmed them so that they would follow the wishes of their masters. Special crystals were placed underground and activated by the sun in battles for supremacy.

Believers claim Atlantean civilization fell because of crystal misuse. Some of the Atlanteans escaped to Egypt, where they built the pyramids using crystal lasers. They also created crystal skulls containing memory banks of information waiting to be decoded.[4]

CLAIMS FOR (UNVERIFIED)

Quartz crystals can be used for healing all ailments and diseases. This is done by using the crystals to create balance in the crystalline structure of the body. By affecting the life force and aura, disease causes the electromagnetic alignment of the life force to become disarranged. Crystals will rearrange the polarity of the life force, thus restoring health.

In addition to utilizing the crystals in special formations, they can also be submerged in pure water, creating a special healing water which should be consumed before programming other crystals or using them to heal ailments.

The body is divided into "chakras" or energy systems. There are seven energy systems in the body which form a synchronized life force through which energy can flow. These chakras are:

- root chakra
- lower abdomen or spleen chakra

- solar plexus chakra
- heart chakra
- throat chakra
- third eye chakra
- crown chakra

Healing is a three-step process that involves clearing blocked energies that impede growth, infusing positive healing energies, and expanding spiritual awareness through your higher self. This involves clearing negative thoughts and eliminating the attitudes that cause those negative thoughts.

CLAIMS AGAINST
None; however, the user of crystal healing should be cautioned not to abandon all other prescriptions, medications, or diets for an unproven cure.

Homeopathic Therapy

Homeopathic medicine was developed by an eighteenth-century chemist, Samuel Hahnemann. During a series of investigative tests of commonly used medicinal substances, he noticed that the standard prescription of the day for malaria was quinine. This surprised him since quinine was a relatively weak astringent compared to others which were available.

To determine what the effects of quinine were, Hahnemann took it himself. To his surprise, his symptoms were those of a malaria sufferer. He continued his tests on healthy individuals by administering other substances to them and observing their symptoms. He noted that not everyone reacted to the substances in the same manner, and he assigned descriptions to the symptoms. The most common symptoms became first-line, less common symptoms were second-line, and the rare symptoms became third-line.

He then went further with his testing and interviewed actual patients who were suffering from various illnesses. By identifying first, second and third line symptoms from these patients, he was able to match the drug description with the illness description. This drug was then the cure for the illness, since it caused the same symptoms if administered to a healthy person.

Hahnemann discovered that the treatment would cause the illness to get worse for a short period of time before the patient began to recover. To avoid this effect, which he called aggravation, he began to dilute his remedies. He discovered that the diluted remedies seemed more effective than the full-strength remedy, and the more dilute the remedy, the more potent it became.

CLAIMS FOR

Homeopathic medicines allow the body to use self-healing to correct problems rather than reactive healing caused by allopathic remedies.

Preparations for seasonal allergies, such as Pollen 30CH and Thymuline 9CH (made from the main pollens found in Canadian trees and grasses), provide relief from allergies.

In 1986, *The Lancet* published a research article based on the studies of Dr. Taylor Reilly who used a double-blind placebo-controlled test to determine the effects of the allergy preparation. The test used 144 patients with active hay fever. Patients treated with the homeopathic medication showed a reduced need for antihistamines and a greater improvement than those treated with the placebo. Dr. Reilly stated that the results of the pilot study could not support the concept that the observed effects were entirely due to the placebo effect, even though the drugs were diluted to the point where, theoretically, none of the original material could remain.

In 1991, the *British Medical Journal* published the results of a review of 107 controlled trials using homeopathic medicines. Dr. Jos Kleijnen and colleagues at the University of Limburg in the Netherlands determined that of 105 trials with interpretable results, 81 showed positive results.

Some conditions which can be treated with homeopathic medicines include:

• acne
• eye dryness
• allergic rhinitis
• physical fatigue
• cankers
• PMS
• conjunctivitis
• rheumatic pain
• coughs
• rhinitis
• diarrhea
• sinusitis
• dysmenorrhea
• sore throat
• dyspepsia

- teething pain
- excess weight
- varicose veins
- warts

CLAIMS AGAINST

The dilution process for the homeopathic medicines has not changed. A mother substance is prepared by grinding or macerating it and dissolving it into a solvent. One drop of the mother substance is added to either 9 drops (decimal dilution or DH) or 99 drops of solvent (centesimal dilution or CH). This would yield a 1DH or 1CH substance. The ingredients are vigorously mixed and diluted again and again.

For example, a 30CH mixture has been diluted 30 times at a ratio of 1:100 and is considered more potent than a 6CH solution. Since this dilution continually reduces the concentration of the original substance, it is estimated that by the time dilution reaches 12CH, less than one mole of the original substance remains. This means that once the 12CH level is passed, none of the original substance remains in solution.

In an article in *The Canadian Medical Association Journal* Dr. Peter Morgan noted that almost two hundred years after the initiation of homeopathic medicine, there is still no scientific support for the theory or evidence that the drugs will perform as suggested.

While there is no proof that homeopathy medicine actually works, at least it is not harmful so as long as people do not forsake consulting with a physician or pharmacist who is trained in homeopathic medications.

Network Chiropractic

Network Chiropractic combines forceful movement of the vertebrae with subtle body energy modifications. It is based on the theory that life-force expression is a combination of the mind, the body, and the energy of the heart. This therapy uses meningeal subluxation combined with the balancing of masculine and feminine forces to create wholeness.

This balance counters "masculine" force with "feminine" kindness. Patients are in balance when they have the inner awareness of when to be assertive and when to be serene. If the vertebrae are not aligned, the heart and its life-force energy cannot effectively balance the masculine-feminine forces and there is no wholeness or harmony.

Patients have the vertebrae forcefully aligned according to standard chiropractic approaches, but they also have gentle, non-forceful pressures applied to the spine to ease and free the life-force flow through the system.

CLAIMS FOR (UNVERIFIED)
When you accept your wholeness, recognize the gentle, playful nature of the feminine side and the destructive, action-oriented masculine side, harmony and balance will return to the body. The alignment of the spine is an important factor in complete wholeness. This integration of the physical and spiritual will create an environment for good health.

CLAIMS AGAINST
None.

Reflexology

The origin of reflexology can possibly be traced to the ancient Egyptians, based on drawings found in a pyramid showing a person working on another person's feet. Modern reflexology is based on the studies of Dr. William Fitzgerald who discovered that there was a relationship between certain areas of the hands and feet and the rest of the body. These tests were performed in the early twentieth century. These findings have been further refined by Eunice Ingham who in 1938 wrote a book titled *Stories the Feet Can Tell: Stories the Feet Have Told.*

The body is divided into ten sections, called longitudinal zones. These zones extend to the hands and feet, providing terminals for treating any medical problems within each zone. This is called zone therapy.

CLAIMS FOR (UNVERIFIED)
By stimulating reflex points in the hands and feet, reflexology can cure chronic back pain and joint disorders and make the nervous system stronger and healthier. In addition, it can make the internal organs and the lymph system healthier.

CLAIMS AGAINST
None.

Notes

CHAPTER 2 / CLINIC THERAPIES

1   "Unproven Methods of Cancer Management: Antineoplastins," *Cancer Association* 33:1 (1983): 57-59.

2   "Cancer Victim Dies Despite Treatment at Radical Clinic," *The Sun*, 18 Dec. 1982, sec. A.

3   H. B. K. Silver, Memorandum on Antineoplastins to Cancer Control Agency of B.C. Library (Vancouver), (1981): Search file 983.

4   M. Dunlop, *Understanding Cancer: An Invaluable Book for Cancer Patients and their Families,* (Toronto: Irwin, 1985), 99-101.

5   H. B. K. Silver, Memorandum on Chacon Cancer Cure to CCABC Library (Vancouver), (1986): Search file 2079.

6   "Unproven Methods of Cancer Management: Hariton Alivizatos, M.D. (Greek Cancer Cure)," *CA* 33 (1983): 252-254.

7   H. B. K. Silver, Memorandum on Greek Cure to CCABC Library (Vancouver), (1986): Search file 705.

8   Brochure, Immunology Research Foundation.

9   "Isolation of Human T-lymphotropic Virus Type III/lymphadenopathy-associated Virus from Serum Proteins Given to Cancer Patients—Bahamas," *Morbidity and Mortality Weekly Report* 34(1985): 489-491.

10   G. A. C. Curt, "Warning on Immunoaugmentative Therapy," Letter to *New England Journal of Medicine* 311, no. 13 (1984): 359.

11   *MMWR* 1984;1985.

12   A. Dlesk et al., "Unconventional Arthritis Therapies," Letter to *Arthritis and Rheumatism* 25, no. 9 (September 1982): 145-146.

13   G. Marchant, "Trick or Treatment?" *Vancouver Magazine* (July 1978): 47.

14   P. Walls, "Healing 'Just a Bunch of Garbage'." *The Province*, 28 Jan. 1982, sec. A-1.

15   J. H. Goldie, "Suggested Agency Policy Regarding 'Simonton

Method' of Treatment for Cancer," *Cancer Control Agency of British Columbia News,* 14 June 1985.

CHAPTER 3 / CHEMICAL THERAPIES

1. "Unproven Methods of Cancer Management: Dimethyl Sulfoxide (DMSO)," *CA* 33, no. 2 (1983): 122-125.

2 "Foods, Drugs or Frauds?" *Consumer Reports* (May 1985): 275-279.

3 J. Gold, "Anabolic Profiles in Late-stage Cancer Patients Responsive to Hydrazine Sulfate," *Nutrition and Cancer* 3 (1981): 13.

4 J. Gold, "Inhibition of Walker 256 Intramuscular Carcinoma in Rate by Administration of Hydrazine Sulfate," *American Society of Clinical Oncology* 25 (1971): 66-71.

J. Gold, "Inhibition of Hydrazine Sulfate and Various Hydrazides, of *in vivo* Growth of Walker 256 Intramuscular Carcinoma, B-16 Melanoma, Murphy-Sturm Lymphosarcoma and L-1210 Solid Leukemia," *Oncology* 27 (1973): 69-80.

J. Gold, "Use of Hydrazine Sulfate in Advanced Cancer Patients: Preliminary Results," *Proceedings of the American Association for Cancer Research and The American Society of Clinical Oncology* 15 (1974): 83.

5 "Unproven Methods of Cancer Management: Hydrazine Sulfate," *CA* 26 (1976): 108-110.

6 M. Ochoa, R. E. Witter, and I. H. Krakoff, "Trial of Hydrazine Sulfate (NSC - 150014) in Patients With Cancer," *Cancer Chemists Report* 59 (1975): 109-118.

7 V. A. Filov and T. M. Burova, "Gluconeogenesis During Therapy of Experimental Tumors With Hydrazine Sulfate," *Oncology* 25 (1971): 66-71.

8 S. S. Mirvish et al., "Comparative Study of Lung Carcinogenesis, Promoting Action in Leukaemo-genesis and Initiating Action in Skin Tumorigenesis by Urethane, Hydrazine and Related Compounds," *International Journal of Cancer* 4 (1969): 318-326.

9 *Ibid.*

10 M. M. Menon and S. V. Bhide, "Perinatal Carcinogenicity of Isoniazid (INH) in Swiss Mice," *Journal of Cancer Research and Clinical Oncology* 105, no. 3 (1983): 258-61.

11   L. Levi et al., "Laetrile: A Study of its Physicochemical and Biochemical Properties," *Canadian Medical Association Journal* 92 (1965): 1057.

12   D. S. Martin et al., "Ineffective Cancer Therapy: A Guide for the Layperson." *Journal of Clinical Oncology* 1 (1983): 154-163.

13   *Ibid.*

14   C. G. Moertel et al., "A Clinical Trial of Amygdalin (Laetrile) in the Treatment of Human Cancer," *N. Eng. J. Med.* 06 (1982): 201-206.

15   *Ibid.*

16   D. M. Greenberg, "The Case Against Laetrile: The Fraudulent Cancer Remedy," *Cancer* 45 (1980): 799-807.

17   *Ibid.*

18   Moertel et al., "A Clinical Trial of Amygdalin (Laetrile) in the Treatment of Human Cancer," 201-206.

19   J. P. Davignon, L. A. Trissel, and L. M. Kleinman, "Pharmaceutical Assessment of Amygdalin (Laetrile) Products," *Cancer Treatment Reports* 62 (1978): 99-104.

20   Greenberg, "The Case Against Laetrile: The Fraudulent Cancer Remedy." 799-807.

21   Schmidt et al., "Laetrile Toxicity Studies in Dogs," *Journal of the American Medical Association* 239 (1978): 943-947.

22   Greenberg, "The Case Against Laetrile: The Fraudulent Cancer Remedy," 799-807.

23   L. Sadoff, K. Fuchs, and K. Hollander, "Rapid Deaths Associated With Laetrile Ingestion," *JAMA* 239 (1978):1532.

24   R. D. Montgomery, "The Medical Significance of Cyanogen in Plant Foodstuffs," *American Journal of Clinical Nutrition* 17 (1965): 103-113.

25   C. Fenselan, S. Pallante, and R. P. Batzinger, "Mandelonitrile B-glucoside: Synthesis and Characterization," *Science* 198 (1977): 625-627.

26   "Death of a Woman, 42, Linked to Laetrile: Coroner Finds Cyanide Poisoning from Massive Doses of Drug," *The Los Angeles Times*, 8 Feb. 1979.

27 "Tumors Grow: Laetrile Kills Lab Test Rats," *The Vancouver Sun,* 5 July 1979.

28 J. D. Herbert and S. Barret, *Vitamins and "Health" Foods: The Great American Hustle,* (Philadelphia: George F. Stickley, 1984), 112.

29 D. S. Martin et al., "Laetrile—A Dangerous Drug," *CA* 27 (1977): 301-304.

30 L. H. Kedda, Personal Communication to CCABC Library, 1978 (Search File 498).

31 C. Aston, Personal Communication to CCABC Library, 1978 (Search File 2001).

32 J. Van Brunt, "Alfacell's Cancer Cure: Hope or Hype?" *Bio/technology* 3, no. 9 (1985): 770-772.

33 R. A. Greenwald et al., "Tetracyclines Inhibit Synovial Collagenase *in vivo* and *in vitro,*" *J. Rheumatol.* 14 (1987): 28.

    F. C. Breedveld et al., "Minocycline Treatment for Rheumatoid Arthritis: An Open Dose Finding Study," *J. Rheumatol.* 17 (19909): 43.

    W. E. Hauser and J. S. Remington, "Effect of Antibiotics on the Immune Response," *Am. J. Med.* 72 (1982): 711-716.

    Daniel J. McCarty, *Arthritis and Allied Conditions* (Philadelphia: Lea & Febiger, 1989).

    W. N. Kelley et al., *Textbook of Rheumatology* (Philadelphia: W. B. Saunders Company, 1993).

CHAPTER 4 / DIETARY THERAPIES

1 B. B. Bowman et al., "Macrobiotic Diets for Cancer Treatment and Prevention," *Journal of Clinical Oncology* 2 (1984): 702-711.

2 "Unproven Methods of Cancer Management: Macrobiotic Diets," *CA* 34 (1984): 60-63.

3 Bowman et al., "Macrobiotic Diets for Cancer Treatment and Prevention," 720-711.

4 "Unproven Methods of Cancer Management: Macrobiotic Diets," 60-63.

5 *Ibid.*

6 H. F. Stich, M. P. Rosin, and M. O. Vallejera, "Reduction With

Vitamin A and Beta-carotene Administration of Proportion of Micronucleated Buccal Mucosal Cells in Asian Betel Nut and Tobacco Chewers," *Lancet* 1 (1984): 1204-1206.

7   G. Hislop, Memorandum on Diet and Cancer to CCABC Library (Vancouver), 1985. (Search File 231).

8   E. Cameron and L. Pauling, "Ascorbic Acid and the Glycosaminoglycans," *Oncology* 27 (1973):181-192.

9   E. Cameron and A. Campbell, "The Orthomolecular Treatment of Cancer II. Clinical Trial of High-dose Ascorbic Acid Supplements in Advanced Human Cancer," *Chemico-Biological Interactions* 9 (1974): 285-315.

10   E. Cameron, A. Campbell, and T. Jack, "The Orthomolecular Treatment of Cancer III. Reticulum Cell Sarcoma: Double Complete Regression Induced by High-dose Ascorbic Acid Therapy," *Chem. Biol. Interactions* 11 (1975):387-393.

11   E. Cameron and L. Pauling, "Supplemental Ascorbate in the Supportive Treatment of Cancer: Reevaluation of Prolongation of Survival Times in Terminal Human Cancer," *Proceedings of the National Academy of Science USA* 75 (1978): 4532-4538.

12   L. J. Loescher and K. A. Sauer, "Vitamin Therapy for Advanced Cancers," *Oncology Nursing Forum* 11 (1984): 38-45.

13   C. R. Arnold, "Megavitamin Therapy," *British Columbia Medical Journal* 22, no. 4 (1980): 126.

14   Loescher and Sauer, "Vitamin Therapy for Advanced Cancers," 38-45.

15   E. T. Creagan et al., "Failure of High-dose Vitamin C (ascorbic acid) Therapy to Benefit Patients with Advanced Cancer: A Controlled Trial," *N. Eng. J. Med.* 301 (1979): 687-690.

16   L. Pauling, "Vitamin C Therapy of Advanced Cancer," *N. Eng. J. Med.* 302 (1980): 694.

17   C. G. Moertel et al., "High Dose Vitamin C Versus Placebo in the Treatment of Patients with Advanced Cancer Who Have Had No Prior Chemotherapy," *N. Eng. J. Med.* 312 (1985): 137-141.

18   C. D. Evans and J. H. Lacey, "Toxicity of Vitamins: Complications of a Health Movement," *British Medical Journal* 292 (1986): 509-510.

19   B. A. Schaywitz et al., "Megavitamins for Minimal Brain Dysfunction: A Potentially Dangerous Therapy," *JAMA* 238 (1977): 1749-53.

20   "Toxic Effects of Vitamin Overdose," Medical Letter 1983;26(667):72-74

      A. Berger and H. Schaumberg, "More on Neuropathy from Pyridoxine Abuse," *N. Eng. J. Med.* 311, no. 15 (1984): 986-987.

      H. Schaumberg et al., "Sensory Neuropath from Pyridoxine Abuse," *N. Eng. J. Med.* 309, no. 8 (1983): 445-53.

21   T. Harada et al., "Effects of Vitamin C on Tumor Induction by Dimethylnitrosamine in the Respiratory Tract of Hamsters Exposed to Cigarette Smoke," *Cancer Letter* 25 (1985): 163-169.

22   "Vitamin Supplements," *Medical Letter on Drugs and Therapeutics* 3 (1984): 66-68.

      N. M. Ellison, "Vitamin C and Cancer." *Cancer Bulletin* 37, no.3 (1985): 117-8.

23   "Toxic Effects of Vitamin Overdose," 72-74.

CHAPTER 5 / HERBAL THERAPIES

1   "Unproven Methods of Cancer Treatment: Chaparral Tea," *CA* 20 (1970): 112-113.

2   I. Hirino, M. Hideki, and H. Masanobu, "Carcinogenic Activity of *Symphytum officinale*," *Journal of the National Cancer Insti tute* 61 (1978): 865-868.

      I. Hirino et al., "Induction of Hepatic Tumors in Rats by Senkirkine and Symphatine," *Journal of the National Cancer Institute* 63 (1979): 469-471.

3   P. M. Ridker et al., "Hepatic Veno-occlusive Disease Associated With the Consumption of Pyrrolizidine-containing Dietary Supplements," *Gastroenterology* 88 (1985):1050-1054.

4   K. J. R. Wightman, *Canadian Medical Association Journal* 117 (1977): 1069.

5   J. D. Sproul, "Communication on Essiac," (Ottawa: Health and Welfare Canada, Health Protection Branch, 1987), CCABC Library Search File 1961E.

6   T. Tenbayashi, "Enhancement of the Host-resistance by *Panax ginseng," Third International Symposium on Detection and Prevention of Cancer* (1976): 242.

7   T. K. Yun et al., *Cancer Detection and Prevention* 6 (1983): 515-525.

8   Y. H. Jie et al., "Immunomodulatory Effects of *Panax ginseng* in the Mouse," *Agents and Actions* 15, nos. 3-4 (1984): 386-91.

9   V. E. Tyler, *The Honest Herbal,* (Philadelphia: George F. Stickley, 1982), 106-110.

10 R. P. Hogan, "Hemorragic Diathesis Caused by Drinking an Herbal Tea," *JAMA* 249 (1983): 2679-2680.

11 C. R. Kumana et al., "Herbal Tea Induced Hepatic Veno-occlusive Disease: Quantification of Toxic Alkaloid Exposure in Adults," *Gut* 26 (1985): 101-104.

12 M. Feigen, "Fatal Veno-occlusive Disease of the Liver Associated With Herbal Tea Consumption and Radiation," *Australia and New Zealand Journal of Medicine* 14 (1984): 61-62.

13 B. E. Haynes et al., "Oleander Tea: Herbal Draught of Death," *Annals of Emergency Medicine* 14, no. 4 (1985): 350-353.

14 K. N. V. Vesselinovitch et al., "Transplacental and Lactational Carcinogenesis by Saffrole." *Cancer Research* 39 (1979): 4378-4380.

15 J. B. Block et al., "Early Clinical Studies With Lapachol (NSC-11905)," *Cancer Chemotherapy Report.* 4, nos. 2, 4 (1974): 27-28.

16 R. K. Morrison et al, "Oral Toxicology Studies with Lapachol," *Toxicology and Applied Pharmacology* 17 (1970): 1-11.

CHAPTER 6 / MISCELLANEOUS THERAPIES

1   K. C. Srivastava and T. Mustafa, "Ginger (*Zingiber officinale*) in Rheumatism and Musculoskeletal Disorders," *Medical Hypotheses* 39, no. 4 (December 1992): 342-3488.

2   S. Thorat and S. Dahanukar, "Can We Dispense With Ayurvedic Samskaras?" *Journal of Postgraduate Medicine* 37, no. 3 (July 1991): 157-1599.

3   R. W. Keen et al., "Indian Herbal Remedies for Diabetes as a Cause of Lead Poisoning," *Postgraduate Medical Journal*, 70, no. 820 (February 1994): 113-114.

4   Judith Larkin, "Counseling With Crystals," in *Newcastle Guide to Healing with Crystals*, eds. Jonathon Pawlik and Pamela Chase, (North Hollywood, CA.: Newcastle Publishing Company Inc., 1988).

Index

Aflatoxin B$_1$, 101
Agpaoa, Tony, 44
AIDS, 41
Alexander technique, 119
Alfacell, 63-64
Alivizatos, Hariton, 36-37
Allantoin, 90
Almonds, 58-59, 107
Aloe vera, 108
American Cancer Society, 29, 37, 48, 49, 55, 75, 90, 109
Ames salmonella lyphimurium test, 62
Amino acid, 35
Aminotransferase, 85
Ampicillin, 66
Amygdalin, 58, 59, 60, 61, 62
Anaphylactic shock, 76, 107
Angioedema, 76
Anise, 93, 94, 95
Anthroposophy, 109
Anticoagulant, 83, 84
Antimicrobial drugs, 66-67
Antineoplastins, 27-29
Antioxidant micronutrients, 78
Apples, 107, 108
Apricots, 58, 107
Arrhythmia, 58, 84
Arteriosclerosis, 112
Arthritis, 18, 22, 23, 24, 30, 41-43, 54, 64, 65, 66, 67, 71, 72, 94, 95, 99, 108, 114, 121
Ascorbic acid, 78, 79
Asthma, 76, 112
Athens Medical Society, 36
Atlantis University, 63
Ayurvedic medicine, 120-122

B

Bacteria, 30, 40, 55, 61, 66, 83
Banting Institute, 98
Bell, Alan W., 64
Beta-carotene, 73, 78
Beta-glucosidase, 59, 61, 62
Betel, 78
Bile duct, 33
Biofeedback, 44, 120
Biomedical Center, 102
Blackwort, 90
Bloating, 76
Bronchitis, 91, 112
Budd-Chiari syndrome, 93
Burdock root, 95, 106
Burton, Lawrence, 38-41
Burzynski, Stanislaw, 27-29
Buzzard gastric juice, 63

C

Cachexia, 56
Cafestol, 33, 35
Caisse, Rene, 95-98
Calcium, 34, 76, 83
Callawaya, 112
Cameron E., 79
Camomile (chamomile), 107
Camphor, 99, 110
Cancers
    bladder, 28
    breast, 28, 61, 62, 78
    bone, 53
    cervical, 78
    colorectal, 78, 81
    esophageal, 78, 104
    leukmia, 36, 37, 39, 96, 100, 112
    liver, 60, 92, 95, 110, 111
    lung, 58, 61, 73, 78, 89, 101
    oral, 78, 79

ovarian, 39, 105
pancreatic, 78
prostate, 39, 57, 74
skin, 61
small-cell histolytic lymphoma, 39
stomach, 78
Captopril, 65
Carcinogens, 58, 62, 79, 80, 82, 83, 92, 101
Cardiac glycosides, 58, 62, 106
Carotenoids, 78
Cassava, 107
Ceftriaxone, 66
Chacon Cancer Cure, 29-31
Chakra, 120
Chamomile, 107
Chapparal, 89-90
Chemicals, 15, 21, 24, 32, 43, 58, 78, 99, 106, 121
Chemotherapy, 55, 59, 74, 75, 81, 90, 105
Cherries, 107
Choke cherries, 107
Cholestatic jaundice, 85
Choline/methionine, 78
Choriocarcinoma, 89
Chuifong Toukuwan, 108
Cisretinoic acid, 65
Coffee enemas, 31, 32, 33, 34, 35, 54
Colitis, 112
Comfrey, 90-92
Compositae, 98, 105, 107
Copper bracelets, 22
Cortisone, 43, 108
Coumarins, 104
Creosote, 89
Crystals, 122-124
Cyanide poisoning, 62, 107

D
Dapsone, 65
Deblocking protein, 39
Degenerative Disease Medical Center, 54
Devil's claw root, 107
Diarrhea, 76, 84, 91, 106, 126, 108
Dietary supplements, 73
Diethylstilbestrol, 78
Digitoxin, 106
Dimethyl benzanthracene, 101
Dimethyl sulfoxide, 53-55
Dioscorides of Anazarbos, 59
Diplomat Tours, 44
DMSO, 42, 53-55
Dominican Republic, 64
Douglas, Donald, 48
Drosophila, 38

E
Eczema, 76
Emphysema, 54
Enzymes, 30, 33, 54
Escherichia coli, 41
Essential oils, 93, 94
Essiac, 95-98
Estradiol, 78
Estrogen, 83, 101
Ethylenediaminetetraacetate, 65
Evening primrose, 93, 94

F
Feverfew, 98-99
Fibrositis, 91
Fish oils, 22
Folate, 76
Folic acid, 78
Free radicals, 33, 78
Friedman, Frank, 38

G

Galiau, Gerry, 46
Gamma-linoleic acid, 93-94
Gangrene, 91
Gerson therapy, 31-36
Ginger, 121
Ginseng, 99-102
GLA, 93-94
Glycosaminoglycans, 79
Gold, J., 56
Gout, 91
Greek Cure, 36-37
Green hartin, 111

H

Hahnemann, Samuel, 124
Haloperidol, 65
Harris, John, 38
Harry Hoxsey's herbal tonic,
    102-103
Health Protection Branch, 97
Hepatitis B, 40
Hepatomegaly, 105
Herbal teas, 103-108
Hodgkin's disease, 38
Hogle, Hugh H., 89
Hokkai-Kisso, 113
Holism, 117
Homeopathic, 124-127
Homeopathy, 118
Horsetail, 106
Hoxsey, H., 102
Hydrazine sulfate, 55-58
Hydrogen cyanide, 107
Hypocalcemia, 77
Hypoglycemia, 58
Hypoproteinemia, 34
Hypotension, 58

I

Immune system, 35, 36, 39,
    43, 54, 72
Immunoaugmentative therapy,
    38-41
Indian tobacco, 107
Inductoscopes, 22
Ingham, Wayne, 29
Inkberry, 107
Ipe roxo, 111
Iscador, 108-110
Isoprinoside, 65

J

Jacobs, Stanley, 53
Juniper, 106

K

Kahweol, 33, 35
Kassell, Robert, 38
Knitbone, 90
Krebs, Ernest, 59
Kusan, Stephanie, 29

L

Lactone, 99
Laetrile, 58-62
Lapachic acid, 111
Lapachol, 111
Leroi, Rita, 108
Leukemia, 36, 37, 39, 96, 100,
    112
Licorice root, 107
Life Extension Products, 55
Linoleic acid, 93, 94
Lymphocyte, 101
Lymphoma, 39
Lymphosarcoma, 89

M

Macrobiotic diets, 73-77
Mandrake root, 101
Manila, 44
Mastitis, 91
Megadose vitamin therapy, 77-85
Mejias, Fernando Chacon, 29
Melanoma, 89
Melilot, 104
Memorial Sloan-Kettering Cancer Center, 56
Menometrorrhagia, 104
Mental illness, 54
Mental imaging, 47
Metabolic therapy, 54
Methadone, 37
Methodist Hospital in Philadelphia, 74
Mexican arthritis treatments, 41-43
Micranthum, 110
Miller, Mildred, 54
Mineral oil, 122
Mistletoe, 108
Moertel, Charles, 59, 81
Monkshood, 121
Morphine, 37
Mussel extract, 22
Mycoplasma infection, 66

N

National Cancer Institute, 40, 59, 63, 90, 98
Naturopathy, 118
Nerioside, 106
Nerium oleander, 105
Network Chiropractic, 128
Niacin, 84-85
Nicotine, 106
Nicotinic acid, 37, 84

Nocardia asteroides, 41
Nordihydroguaiaretic acid, 90
Nutmeg, 106

O

Oleander, 106
Oleandrin, 106
Oleandroside, 106
Oncogenes, 27
Oregon Health Science University, 53
Orthomolecular therapy, 77
Oshawa, George, 73
Otitis, 91
Oxygenators, 32

P

Palcossio 55, 63
Palencia, M.A., 63
Panax ginseng, 99
Panax pseudoginseng, 99
Panax quinquefolium, 99
Pannon, 63-64
Papilledema, 82
Parthenolide, 99
Pauling, L., 79, 81
Peaches, 58, 107
Pears, 107
Pectin, 22
Penicillamine, 65
Pennyroyal oil, 107
Peppermint tea, 107
Pepsin, 32, 92
Percodan, 37
Pharmacological therapy, 64-66
Philippine Medical Association, 45
Philippines, 43
Placebo, 17, 18, 36, 45, 61, 81, 95, 96, 97, 125
Plums, 107

Pokeweed, 107
Polypeptides, 28
Positive imaging, 47
Procaine hydrochloride, 55
Psoriasis, 105
Psychic surgery, 43-46
Pulmonary hemorrhages, 91
Pyrethrins, 99
prithioxine, 65
Pyrrolizidine alkaloids, 92

R

Radiation therapy, 29, 59, 74
Radon, 22
Red ginseng, 102
Red lapacho, 111
Reflexology, 129
Reserpine, 101
Resperin Corporation, 95
Retinoids, 78
Rheumatoid arthritis, 22, 41,
    64, 66, 67, 95, 121
Riboflavin, 76
Rickets, 76
Rifamycin, 66
Rottino, Antonio, 38
Royal College of Physicians and
    Surgeons, 96
Russian Comfrey, 90

S

Safrole, 110, 111
Saint Barnabas Medical Center, 71
Sassafras, 110-111
Sattilaro, Anthony J., 74
Schramm, Henning, 108
Scopolamine, 101
Scurvy, 76
Selenium, 78
Senkirkine, 92
Septicemia, 29

Shave grass, 106
Siegel, 101
Simonton Method, 47-49
Simonton, Carl O., 47
Snake venom, 22
Society for Cancer Research,
    108
Solarama boards, 22
Staphylococcus aureus, 41
Star anise, 110
Steiner, Rudolf, 108
Steroids, 42
Stich, Hans, 83
Sweet woodruff, 104
Symphatine, 92
Symphytum officinale, 90

T

Tabebuia, 111
Tabebuia altissima, 111
Taheebo, 111-113
Taiguic acid, 111
Tecomin, 111
Terpene, 99
Tetracycline, 66-67
Thalidomide, 65
Thaminase, 106
Thiopyridoxine, 65
Tiopronin, 65
Titerpenoid saponins, 100
Tonka beans, 104
Toxins, 32, 33, 55
Tuberculosis, 31, 43

U

U.S. Food and Drug Adminis-
    tration, 15, 16, 38, 64, 90,
    103, 110
Ulcers, 43, 90, 113
University of Michigan, 28
Urethane, 101

Urticaria, 76

V
Valerian, 113-114
Veno-occlusive disease, 93, 105
Viscum album, 108
Vitamin A, 78, 81-82
Vitamin B, 76
Vitamin B_{12}, 83
Vitamin B_{17}, 59
Vitamin B_6, 82
Vitamin C, 77, 78, 79, 80, 81, 82-83
Vitamin D, 22, 61, 83
Vitamin E, 77, 84, 94
Vitamin K, 84
Vomiting, 76

W
WD40, 22
Weinberger, Marvin I., 108
Wightman, K. J. R., 96
Wolfsbane, 121
Woodruff, 104
Wright, Donald F. & Carol, 44

Y
Yin and yang, 73
Yukon Medical Association, 45

Z
Zinc, 78